BUTTERFLY IN THE WELL

Village Opinions with Exploratory Knack

ROBERT EWING

ISBN 978-1-954345-95-9 (paperback)
ISBN 978-1-954345-97-3 (digital)

Rushmore Press LLC
1 800 460 9188
www.rushmorepress.com

Printed in the United States of America

Choice, not chance, decides destiny

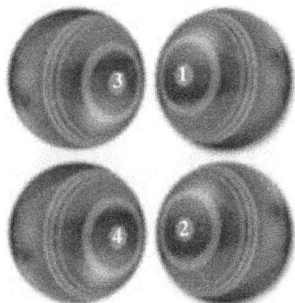

❧ Contents ❧

Life is a journey...

...Home

Generic contents

"In many ways, we are like travelers in a rocket ship
hurtling through space on an unknown trajectory."
G. and *J. Lenski*, Human Societies, 1970 /74

The dynamic content of this work relates the comments to twenty-five subjects posted at website by Village magazine (marketed as: "Ireland's political and cultural magazine"), concerning which there is background historical narrative by me - the principal commentator.

I relate the subjects as I evaluated and responded to each between March 23rd 2016 and February 2nd 2018. And I relate my picture to them (my first school photograph), posted June 28th 2016.

Participation was invited by way of the ideal: "Village promotes in its columns the fair distribution of resources, welfare, respect and opportunity by the investigation and analysis of inequalities, unsustainable development and corruption, and the media's role in their perpetuation; and by acute cultural analysis."

My intention to relate my involvement with Village as a book began August 21st 2016. The title derives from the title of a song by composer John Adorney: "A Butterfly in the Well".

My comments generally concern the failure of secondary school education to relate such studies as published since 1872 relating State component cultural defects, and report the necessity of obtaining State accountability which would challenge such defects as tend to subordinate public policy to prestige and money-culture: "It's the law" the public hears, and: "It's all up here" reasoned father as a civil proceedings lay-litigant, but what is "law"? Its objective is social order and its method is to generate respect for ownership, whether of property or position. "It's all a con" said newspaper reporter to me, and State neglect to educate all to what law is advantages all the predatory routines.

Village wrote and published three consequential topics, and consequently I commented again to subjects nine, eleven and twenty-five. The index states both the subject dates and commentator names.

I also relate the comments to 'thesun.co.uk', at "What was the Aberfan disaster, when did it happen and how many people were killed?" I was reminded of that coal board and school management negligence while collecting the original of my posted picture for this book close to the fiftieth "Trafalgar Day" since – October 21st 1966/2016.

The Joe Cox tragedy occurred during these comments; and I was reminded recently of a written statement to me of three decades ago from a Bedford female student: "god nobody could say you didn't try and warn me."

"His written work [aged eight] is of sound imaginative content."

The concluding chapter relates parts of the reply to me from Ian Jones, and (with the exception of the full-stop after "Griffon" and concluding question-mark, for example), is as it developed and concluded prior to his response.[1]

"Robert [aged nine] can write a very interesting composition."

"Marbles" at school was the task of lodging one's marble in the brick-size gap at the base of the school-building, and/or dislodging opponent marble/s.

"His contributions to class-work [aged eleven] often prove invaluable." /"He is usually a most effervescent member of his tutor group."

Our class visited the local manor buildings, at which I independently measured wall widths. On return, the teacher offered the class an opportunity to relate any aspect of the visit, and I stood up and related my survey.

I relocated a field-to-field gateway while visiting Ireland, as would [the Irish Management Institute:] "a friendly outside eye on the company's [the community's] activities."

"He [aged fourteen] fully deserves his [history class] position." /"A friendly, helpful member of the tutor group."

There are nine more pictorial 'marbles'; junior-school pupils at the "India" face of the Phoenix Park monument, as if "Marchington" (behind "Wellington"); father celebrating his sixty-sixth birthday relative to discovering the village called "Ireland"; "Christ College Farm" house (sketched for the "Village" part of my geography project), shown relative to the butterfly postage-stamp: "Aglais urticae", as 'paying one's last respects' to copyright; my parents-to-be (with one of mother's cousins); my first home; the village school (my youngest brother

---

[1]   Such as here too, I wrote: "very interesting" (a quotation related on this page thus immediately subsequent to "response."), prior to him replying: "Very interesting…"

faces toward the School Lane elm spinneys); the manor buildings; the false summons pinned to my front door; and a Spitfire over Northern Ireland.

My historical notes include references to three-and-a-half hundred books. And my State component documentation and relevant evidence is as extensive and challenging to relate comprehensively and concisely: "Munich. Of course they had to attack the Agreement after it was made because they attacked everything Chamberlain did or did not do." Indeed, living-off everything the individual did or did not do: "Mr Robert Ewing may be mistaken as to the manner in which courts of law seek to attain justice." The public is lived-off, and the methods of the predatory routines must be comprehensively debated: "judges do not believe the [justice] minister concerned with the validity of judgments, and they believe they serve the minister by routinely following the chief State solicitor who, it seems, routinely opposes litigation against the State."

"He [aged fifteen] willingly gave up a Saturday morning to participate [at school] in a CSE standardisation meeting." /"He has an intelligent [artist] approach."

"Potter's bar" is not meant read as a poem…

Preambulary introduction

"Even worse, we have only the most limited knowledge
of the vehicle – our society – on which our lives depend."
Gerhard and *Jean Lenski*, Human Societies, 1970 /74

"What an array of attainment and effort grades!"

History may now clarify why a protestant man asked Irish
catholic neighbours to shut his protestant community in a barn
and set light to it.

"He expressed his appreciation for ...certainty and finality
in the matter."

"The vague public mind will appreciate some signal duty
before the precise, occupied administration perceives it."

The "certainty" to avoid, as expressed June 1872; and the
"finality" to avoid, as expressed June 1942:[1]

> "The defects of bureaucracy are, indeed, well known."
> /"It is an inevitable defect, that bureaucrats will care
> more for routine than for results..."

> "'The State' is not a benevolent, white-bearded old
> gentleman, at present sitting on some cloud and waiting
> to be fetched down to earth."

---

[1]   Walter Bagehot /Douglas Reed

"In those circumstances Mr Ewing has reviewed the matter, he has pointed out that this [fire] ...was necessary to obtain certainty. He expressed his appreciation for ['This Torch Freedom'] ... because it did as he said provide certainty and finality". As Kyle parish had said of teacher Elsie Ewing: "the good you have done by your residence amongst us".

Indeed, the protestant man was no sadist; on the contrary, he pursued the signal duty to save the protestant community from the penal code of bureaucratic certainties and State reputation finalities such as Irish catholic too would protest about: "There is no winning with those people"; and such as writers Antony Jay and Jonathan Lynn would relate:

> "I have news." "Yes?" "Do you want the bad news first?" "You mean there's bad news and good news?" "No, there's bad news and worse news."

Thus while June 1872 is news, June 1942 will be a bulletin:

> "A bureaucracy is sure to think that its duty is to augment official power, official business, or official members, rather than to leave free the energies of mankind; it overdoes the quantity of government, as well as impairs its quality."

> "'The State' is that great army of exclusive and exempt and privileged and mutually back-scratching officials which we already have – multiplied by a thousand."

Officialdom indeed; no "good news", just perpetual strife:

"This decision cost the R.A.F. at least a thousand Spitfires which should have been in reserve when the Battle of Britain started."

And a consequence of perpetual strife is reserve:

"Dowding thought nothing of our Air Ministers, from the last war to Sinclair – except Swinton. He said Swinton was ousted by Nuffield (I heard this at the time) and Kingsley Wood, and that is why Kingsley Wood got Swinton's job."

"Chamberlain made up his mind that he must sacrifice me"; "He gave me no warning, he just sent for me and said I must go." "This decision", "to get an easier time in Parliament", "allowed my successor, Sir Kingsley Wood, to take away the great Castle Bromwich factory …from Vickers and give it to Lord Nuffield, which Kingsley Wood did for political reasons, to the dismay of many of the Air Staff."

Thus Chamberlain set light to a "great army" at Castle Bromwich, and to the dismay of many officials?

Reputation would just send for him and say he must go:

"I [of Little Ship Street] caused inquiries to be made[1] with An Garda Síochána ["Do you have any news - any news?"] as to the Plaintiff's whereabouts."

Of capital importance, however, a dashing catholic capitally ordered that the headstone for the burnt community would

---

[1] Evasive response to Robert Ewing such as the minister for justice had undertaken: "I have had enquiries made…"

honour them with the epitaph: 'News no longer local is of
no interest.' Only "officialdom, the implacable enemy of all
human freedom and dignity", would yet confuse even catholic
journalists to regard John McGahern as a dash too critical of the
State:

> "'News no longer local is of no interest.' McGahern
> [wrote the journalist] was writing of …a very weak
> sense of ownership of the State, but a very strong sense
> of local belonging."

That was either critical of dashing Ireland, indeed, or Fintan
O'Toole was a barn-owl writing of his dwelling as an Irish barn-
owl would, in order to hoot not for the "certainty and finality" to
be got from determining "to represent effectually general sense
in opposition to bureaucratic sense", by way of torched barns,
but an exemplary performance of community objectives such as
Village attempts and the State is supposed to reward.

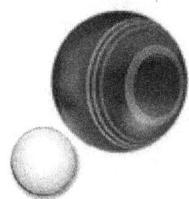

Indeed you are

"This is incredible, in fact unbelievable cheek & nerve
to write something of this kind, knowing the truth."
Robert Ewing concerning the "cornered rat", 1985

"Abbeyville saved my life", concluded my father, William
Ewing.

"To whom are we listening? To the man who took unfair
advantage of his position to influence weaker minds..."[1]
"In fact, I should observe that throughout the entirety of my
relationship with the plaintiff's father I was paid no more than
£900 which I received from ...s [the Supreme Court: "a firm of
solicitors involved in the transaction"] being the balance in his
account, and a further £1,000 being a cheque he had received
from Nenagh Co-op."

A firm of solicitors involved in the transaction?

The Supreme Court: "I would like to add one or two further
observations ...which, for all judges of the superior courts, will
be statements of the obvious."

One or two solicitors involved in the transaction?

"As I have observed, it is certainly the case that the plaintiff's
father was advised to settle these proceedings, [concerning
which the solicitor involved in the transaction lied: "I attended
to give evidence not for one or other party, but as available to

---

[1] Green street courthouse judge, September 1803

both"] and that advice was furnished in the clearest of terms to him by his Senior Counsel".

Meaning "the clearest of terms", such as "both" clients, rather than "one or two"?

"Mr. K...y has behaved totally honourably throughout the entire matter ["Mr. Ewing was my client" /"I at all times regarded Mr. Ewing as my client"] at some considerable expense and trouble to himself".

Any further observations? "Mr. K...y was certainly on the face of it a somewhat reluctant and concerned person who was worried about the level of his existing payments and commitments involved in the contract."

Indeed, one firm of solicitors involved ("not for one or other party, but as available to both" in the transaction - contrary to the Law Society guidelines), and not truly as available to both; just as the supposed non-client, notified that he was registered owner of the entirety of the lands transferred to him, furnished advice to me "in the clearest of terms" which he contradicted in communication with others (while my father was neither notified that the supposed non-client would be registered for the entirety of the lands, nor that he had been registered):

> "Mr. K...y urged him strongly that he was wasting his time building walls etc. at the house, as this place, house and all was going to be sold to him, Mr. K...y. "Your father wants to sell it to me", he said."

> "R-of-way to be protected in any event. Needs guarantee of this as Robert Ewing is raising cane about it."

"To whom are we listening? To the man who took unfair advantage of his position to influence weaker minds..." "I can loan you money if you need it." In court, irrelevantly: "I believe he knew exactly what he had borrowed."

What "he knew", retrospectively, was: "Monies advanced to get a hold of property through debt!!" "Needs guarantee", as effectively I was raising cash; and would advise my father to challenge the harasser's "hold" once his proposal to halve the dwelling was 'to be accepted in any event' as part of the negotiation process. And such was the origin of his litigation: to get a hold of property sought immediately prior to the dispute, "and comprising 3 acres, 0 roods and 39 perches" (the most part of "the lawn"):

> "He made it clear last wk to me, [Robert Ewing] that his proposal regarding the line across the lawn, would not be compromised. That line is unacceptable to me, and I know it is unacceptable to you as regards leaving a realistic environment for the house.
>
> Mr. K...y is completely unaware at present that we can be equally clever, and we should carry on playing the 'fools' until ["his lease runs out"] March."

The unavailability of solicitors to challenge the harassment had thus generated a dispute, for my father was entitled to re-transfer of the dwelling, and the denial of that performance was indeed "unacceptable":

> "A condition is a term of the contract which goes so directly to the root of the contract, or, in other words, is so essential to its very nature, that if the circumstances

are, or become, inconsistent with the condition, all executory obligations under the contract may be treated as discharged by a party who is not in default."

And such was the evidence available to the solicitor:

"Present position is as if I am retransferring to Bill without getting anything for it." /"Would transfer it back to Bill subject to time limit [a reference to £5,000 harassment monies] & r-of-way." /"Proviso that the r-of-way remains."

Contrary to such attendance notes concerning the harasser's attempt to "guarantee" access, and despite such notes being available to co-defendant senior counsel, the harasser would lie at re-hearing that the solicitor could justify his right of way claim:

"I told her [a lie concerning the late Mrs Lennon] that I had purchased the right-of-way with the [adjacent] lands [the first lands which involved the solicitor as the purchaser's solicitor] and that my Solicitor [a reference to "the solicitor" without identifying him] would clarify this for her if she needed clarification."

The clarification I received from the harasser: "I was leaving you with the house because I felt sorry for you." He was referring to his proposal of "paying …a further £1,500 and …releasing …right-of-way …for ownership of that portion of the Lawn marked on the map [almost half the dwelling sought at one-fifth of its "conservative" valuation] and comprising 3 acres, 0 roods and 39 perches". His mistake was not to maintain sufficient confidence toward him; I accepted negotiation with him as concerning co-ownership (guaranteeing the succession), and the re-transfer and debt; but his new solicitor would not invite me to his meeting with my father; such proposals were stealth, and indeed the real proposal was: "a further £1,500", which was the type of deceit which I would warn my father about because of the subsequent attempt to dictate, yet unaware of the proposals – not "a further" owner (a co-owner), but "a further £1,500":

> "I think he is hoping, that now you're gone, you will not come back for some time, & that he can lodge £300 or so in your account and take the lawn for another yr. And subsequently retain possession and his position."

The first judge asked the harasser why he had not re-transferred the dwelling, and received no reply; because the harasser was plaintiff in order to continue attempt to halve the dwelling; "because I felt"? His declarations to me subsequently were: "You are a marked man in this parish", and: "You got involved"; both of which evidently had a pre-dispute origin, as undisclosed correspondence relates:

> "Our client called to see us [the new solicitors] today and expressed concern regarding the behaviour of your Client's son and damage he has caused to the property [re-design of the house begun partly to register that the harasser did not own it; such as subsequently related concerning "possession and his position": "Mr. K...y cannot avoid confirming that the 6½ acres is not his"] and threats he has made concerning same. [the harasser

not only claimed to me that paying "£45,000" meant ownership of the dwelling but subsequently responded to me that he would 'take the lot'; and would many times damage the property with cattle] On this account our Client requires possession of Land Certificate"

"We [the son of the solicitor] note that it is our clients sons behaviour which has given rise to concern on your clients behalf, indeed" /"We now enclose Land Certificate". Subsequently: "I recall a letter from [the new solicitor] …in which he made allegations about Mr. Robert Ewing's actions and I wrote back ["as between Solicitors"] noting that no allegations had been made against our client"

And: "I wrote back noting" was not the first time that he lied that reference to me had no significance as concerned the ownership issue:

"We cannot forward you [William Ewing] Land Certificate as …K…y is now the registered owner of same [registered over three years previously] and as such has possession of the Land Certificate" /"You know very well how …K…y was registered as owner of the lands … He was registered on foot of a contract and transfer signed by you, [by way of the written obligation to "re-convey" the dwelling] the land certificate was handed over to his solicitor [the new solicitor] at his request [thirty-seven weeks previous to this correspondence which involved disclosing the whereabouts of the certificate] as Mr. K…y was the person entitled to ownership of same."

His compliance with the harasser's request for the Land Certificate may have generated the specific attempt to dictate which generated the dispute ("He made it clear [fourteen weeks subsequent to receiving the certificate] …that his proposal …would not be compromised"), and thereby the declaration: "I was leaving you with the house…"

The first litigation was of the routine reference to me which began concerning the right of way controversy, continued concerning the Land Certificate, and continued concerning Land Commission consent (as noted by my co-defendant, who examined the Commission file: "Robert Ewing (son) accused wrongly"), and again continued, after the litigation began as "the same" and further litigation (the 'hearing' of which was initially averted by me, by way of dismissal of the second co-defendant solicitors – the intention of the lawyers being the same as would determine the re-hearing, which was "set up"), and continued after that by way of a false summons, again successfully (just as the proposal to halve the lawn was begun by way of involving me). The further and "same" litigation was attempt to exploit my first initiative to have the second solicitors dismissed; and the third co-defendant solicitors would be dismissed too, in order to obtain first hearing of the litigation, but the judge, at the conclusion of the first hearing (a completed hearing of three days duration), would not conclude his adjudication:

> "Judge Cassidy gave a summing up:
> 'If [the solicitor] …asked Mr. Ewing that in order to sell a portion of land he would have to transfer the whole property in order to get round the Land Commission, Mr. [the solicitor – 'now' a judge of the District Court]

...might have more experience than himself in these matters, but it is my opinion that this might conflict ...as they were not being notified' ...The judge then completed by saying to counsel, 'it may be a case of... (finished in Latin).'

Mr. Ewing gave an undertaking to appoint legal representation."

Thus both judge and solicitor re-directed my father by way of reference to the Land Commission:

"K...y ...feels [three months after "a map" was prepared] that the transfer of same should go ahead straight away. He [sought and obtained alternative maps behind the future vendor's back: "these later maps"] feels that he has substantially paid the greater part of the purchase money for same.

The difficulties I see arising [were not of the map] and this is [not of "a map", indeed, but of "the maps", indeed] that the area in transfer is [the low quality land] substantial and leaves you with an uneconomic holding, with the result that the Land Commission may very well feel that they should acquire the balance of the lands from you. I think this is quite likely to occur as almost half [one third] the holding is going in the present proposed transfer."

Manufactured evidence attendance note: "Mr. Ewing took the map prepared ...with the view to having it revised if..." He did not view any map ("none of these maps were made available"), until he was a co-defendant, and the solicitor already had the "later maps" (received in July, 1982; thus prior to the supposed attendance). "He decided to postpone discussions" ("in the light of what has been discussed on this occasion")? The "proposed transfer" was "agreed" and could "go ahead straight away".

Thus neither the agreed sale concerning the debt, nor the subsequent sale (which the Land Commission might well have stopped, as the harasser already owned rather more land than most locally), and nor the first hearing, had result; re-hearing began six years subsequent to the ordering of discovery after the first hearing, and by means which my co-defendant had alleged prior to co-defendant senior counsel "banging the table" (their second meeting, which like the first was a result of the imminent possibility of hearing): "the delaying tactics of the legal profession".

"Strenuous efforts were made by Senior Counsel to convince the plaintiff's father to settle his claim"; "banging the table to show his displeasure that I [William Ewing] insisted in going into court for the long awaited hearing." Only my co-defendant could not be convinced that he "was wasting his time":

> "The purpose of this meeting was to inform me to settle
> out of court, sell my home to pay legal costs, and accept
> that this whole affair was carried out in such a manner, at
> my bidding. Shocked and outraged at what I was hearing,
> I consequently left the meeting."

A commenter to Village: "note the way the matter is twisted by the official so as to make me appear the villain of the piece."

The official?

"a man whose ambition is to sit at an official desk,
with a pile of forms before him, dressed in a little brief
authority, and there to thwart and harass and bully his
fellow-citizens by every means in his power, which is
unlimited."[1]

"The official response was that it was "not intended as a
threatening comment ...I regret if you felt threatened by this
comment as this was not the intention..." ...a kind-of wriggling
and squirming gobbledegook ...what I "felt" is beside the point."
However, anything the solicitor "felt" was his instructed point:

"I haven't dealt with same [lie concerning reply to an
independent solicitor involved] except to express the
view ...that the letter is libelous of ...K...y.
     Do you wish me to reply in detail to the matter,
[he just had; for example: "K...y has behaved totally
honourably throughout the entire matter at some
considerable expense and trouble"] personally I don't
think I should, ["express" here that I replied "in detail"]
I certainly won't without your instructions."

A subsequent reply to the same solicitor: "we already put his
[William Ewing's] sons view point to him"; the harasser had
since begun to exploit the supposed post-sale so-called loans
("Present position is as if..."), just as the replied to solicitor
had warned my father by way of writing to him eleven weeks
previously. The judge of the District Court was asked for a
written Statement and thus lied:

---

[1]   Douglas Reed, June 1942

"I am quite sure that I warned him [William Ewing]
that ...it was inevitable that he would have to part with
at least part of the farm." Subsequently: "every effort
was made to warn Mr. Ewing in relation to the likely
outcome of his course of conduct but he chose to ignore
this advice."

Again, not the clearest of terms: "quite sure" /"every effort".
And his (the solicitor's) attendance notes are evidence that
no warning occurred, despite various obvious opportunities
concerning the pre-sale agreed 'loans': sale of "part" required
Land Commission consent. In other words, his mention of
Land Commission consent was belated, just as my father noted
concerning the report which claimed to relate my "view point":
"A somewhat belated interest in the Ewing state of affairs!
Written ...only because..." "I am quite sure that I warned him";
effectively concerning the opinion "that he might get the whole
farm back" ("Mr. K...y owned what was precisely half of" the
original "Abbeyville" lands), and despite the "future leasing,
proposed sale of part." Thus "warned" against a supposed
friendship which subsequently he related as: "his course of
conduct" – friendship (or trust) a "course of conduct"? And
the harasser (or untrustworthiness) provided with "a Power of
Attorney to enable Mr. ...K...y to manage affairs in case ...there
was any danger of anybody else intervening in Mr. Lennon's
affairs" (while "Mr. Ewing ...was in constant transit from
Ireland"); "his position", indeed!
    "In December, 1981, he told me that he proposed to sell
part of his lands", and "I am quite sure that I warned him that
at the rate he was drawing ...he would have to part with at

least part" - no warning concerning the Land Commission. "In December, 1982 ["At the time of the contract"] he had already drawn some £19,000 from …K…y" /"already received some £19,000"; £8,000 of which concerned future rent of the land to April 1986, but as my father noted: "no intention re long leasing"; and noted concerning the 'loans' subsequent to "the contract" ('loans' begun as guarantee for part of the sale payment being released which the solicitors had withheld relative to capital acquisitions tax concerns): "Ewing threatened by R...y, [the new solicitor] take the consequences if not willing to settle".

Yet I was unaware of that threat when I advised the dispute: the harasser had 'now' "to settle" or "take the consequences", as the false sale contract sum of £45,000, contrary to what the transfer states, was unpaid.

The "consequences", as ventured by my co-defendant at the first hearing, were that "the contract thus could not be valid". The "consequences", as ventured by co-defendant senior counsel at the re-hearing: a "document" relating false sums (concerning which, at the first hearing: "Mr. Ewing even ventured to ask Mr. K…y whether this [false sum] might be a mistake on the document"), had caused the vendor to be "suspicious" concerning how much sale money was paid. "In fact, I should observe that throughout the entirety …I was paid no more than £900 …and a further £1,000" (that solicitor was evidently paid considerably more than that); and the "no more than" and "further" "consequences" ventured: "I had to pay Senior Counsel and Junior Counsel fees out of my own pocket for these proceedings…" Just as the Supreme Court would lie of the origin of those proceedings, that I "thought that the sale price of the lands ["his father sold land"] was well below the true valuation of the property"; and would lie of the origin of "the existing proceedings" that I had "suspicions" concerning the sale.

The agreed sale price for the land was £35,000; but the transfer of the dwelling meant false sum ("for [immediate] Revenue [Commission] purposes"); only the Court would not relate the two sums in any one judgment, just as the Court would lie just as the harasser wanted to confuse me, that he had bought the land - involving no reference to the "consequences" of that supposed sale: transfer of the dwelling (and not retransferred), and accumulating debt:

> "It is important to stress that the issue was determined once and for all ["the decision of the High Court on appeal from the Circuit Court is final and un-appealable"] irrespective of the arguments made or evidence adduced by either party." /"On the 6th May, 1999, Robert Ewing separately issued High Court proceedings. He sought to re-open the issues which had been determined. William Ewing unfortunately died on the 20th January, 1999."

"It is important to stress": "the legal team did not seem to want my son by my side, and indeed" such attempted thus twice by the Court "once and for all"; "unfortunately" "separately issued", "and indeed I", as "was determined" or "adduced" by neither party, "died on the 20th January, 1999."

And judge Cassidy's disinclination to adjudicate: had he died too?

"The matter was apparently part heard at that time"
[further lie: "but subsequently the Ewings served
another notice of change of solicitors"] /"Thereafter
Judge Cassidy made an order for discovery" /"That order
necessarily resulted in further delay." /"The learned High
Court Judge ["in the existing proceedings"] concluded
his judgment, as he had started it..." /"The plaintiff
expressed concern regarding delay in the delivery of
[oral judgment not provided in writing for almost half
a year] the High Court judgment" /"They ["the same"
proceedings; neither Supreme Court mentioned the
Circuit Court proceedings that only alleged debt] were
part heard at the time of the judges unfortunate death."

The Court lied that "the existing proceedings" concerned
procedural issues subsequent to the appeal hearing relative to the
re-hearing: "the unfavourable result, from the plaintiff's point of
view of those proceedings" /"the "damning bill of costs" that
was directed entirely against his then [three year] ill father."
Anything subsequent to the said appeal (including "ill father")
was irrelevant to the proceedings which repeated Circuit Court
claims, and to the various legal professional defendants; such
was the Court's reference to "history":

> "In the following years [to the contract and transfer - "the
> events which took place in 1982 and 1983"] it is clear
> [exploitation of the second of "the same" proceedings]
> that the relationship ["between" the harasser and "the
> Ewings"] ...was very unhappy."

To whom are we listening?

The future bar association president involved with the negligence panel (the third co-defendant) solicitors:

> "In more recent times [the second co-defendant solicitors were dismissed] relationships between the parties have been far from good and ...the [Circuit Court] plaintiff issued second Equity Civil Bill proceedings" /"In reality the 2 equity proceedings are the same"

Since the "relationships between the parties" had not been "far from good", what was the nature of the second of "the same" proceedings, but the first? To whom, or to what, are we listening: "a sting"? Just as the Court would not state "the trust", and indeed lied: "a trust", as concerned my father's involvement with the solicitor and harasser; because the law requires the clearest of terms for striking out proceedings:

> "The case against the four solicitors is nowhere clearly stated." ["The case" varied "against the four solicitors", and was "clearly stated"] /"Robert Ewing was attempting to reopen the issue raised by his father in the counterclaim in the Circuit Court proceedings and to combine with it allegations of negligence, and indeed fraud, by the four firms of solicitors who did at different times act for Mr Ewing Senior, in relation to his dispute with Mr K...y." /"He believes that the conduct of the Defendants or, at least some of them, was to say the least, suspect and..." /"was firmly but delicately rejected"

And since lies do not constitute clear case for dismissal, and since that first High Court litigation necessarily involved repeat of the prior claim against the harasser, I subsequently had to litigate against the State itself. And that would not be "firmly but delicately rejected", rather an aggressive defence strategy began to have the litigation struck-out, and the Supreme Court again lied, rather than relate the conflict:

> "Mr. Ewing is clearly deeply concerned about the events which took place in 1982 and 1983." /"The issues raised here are ones which have been ruled on in earlier decisions and have been supplemented by actions against the many lawyers engaged and involved." /"he combined these claims with allegations of negligence and fraud against [quoted case-law: "with actions against the lawyers who have acted for or against the litigant in earlier proceedings"] …a number of solicitors firms, who, at various times, had acted for (or against) the family."

Involving "the four solicitors" had provided the High Court with immediate access to each concerning the mistreatment alleged, and as defendants, rather than as witnesses, that process could only help clarify whether or not there was "cause of action" against the harasser, who evidently throughout his relation to my father exploited the non-availability of solicitors, and evidently specifically exploited the non-availability of co-defendant senior counsel at the re-hearing. The new solicitor was immediately responsible for the "damning bill of costs" (and his client was rightly held to account for it, not indeed the client's solicitor):

> "The matter was further delayed [affidavit lies: "instructed three …and dismissed each" of the first

three solicitors; "revoked ...instructions to the Third Firm ...when ...about to be listed ...for hearing in January 1990" – "listed for ...March 1990 ...but I was informed ...February ...that their instructions had been withdrawn" – contradicting: "when ...listed ...for ... January"] and complicated by the frequent changes of solicitors and counsel by the defendants and by the defendants representing themselves."

The Court, as was routine with the various lawyers, would state nothing both accurate and significantly relevant about the dispute and litigation:

"The Circuit Court made a declaration [an order] he [the harasser] was entitled to the right of way [the Court knew that judge Cassidy had declared against the right of way claim] which he claimed."

And the minister for justice had also been somewhat "beside the point": "I have had enquiries made in the Land Registry"; relevant "enquiries" would have been at the Law Society (as the solicitor was 'now' a judge of the District Court, and as such could be dismissed by the government).

"I should state", lied the fourth solicitor; and the minister was as deceitful: "I should also point out that the Judiciary are independent in the exercise of their judicial functions, subject only to the Constitution and the law." /"This appears to be a civil matter and as such it is outside the scope of my official functions to intervene in any way. It is also outside the scope of my official functions to give legal advice ["a sting", indeed] ...or to offer comment in relation to any particular Court proceedings."

In other words, the enquiry procedure provided to the public
is "statements of the obvious" based (a lie for most eventualities,
such as the solicitor had, irrespective of the relevant logic; for
example: "That's a typing error"), and litigation procedure is the
same; the routine is to resist allegation or litigation against State
component; and such is routine pretence of law availability:

> "We [the solicitor] overlooked when we were writing
> to you [William Ewing] drawing your attention to the
> position in relation to the succession act of 1965. We
> have not discussed this end of the matter yet with Mr.
> Lennon but we will of course have to discuss it with
> him" /"I don't think Mr. Lennon would be claiming his
> rights under the …Act but I think he probably wants
> some concession in relation to the money and stock…"
> Subsequently: "and he is agreeable I think to accept this"
> /"I think this would be to your benefit in the sense…"

"That reads to me as a kind-of wriggling and squirming
gobbledegook with a sting in its tail. For note" that my father
was referred to as if he might have influenced a "weaker"
mind. Yet he was disinclined to either discern that a "written
threat" was involved, or challenge it; he was not quite aware that
legal professionals are particularly inclined to refer to money,
and particularly specialise in threats; the threats concerning
money would have to go too far before he could discern them as
methods, thus: "Rubbish" /"Land Commission used as threat".

"I regret if you felt threatened…" /"what I "felt" is beside the
point." "Counsel [for the plaintiff] inferred that Mr. [William]
Ewing was afraid of his son" (fear generated by threats: solicitor
routine); "Mr. Ewing replied that he wouldn't be afraid of any

of his sons." "Mr. Ewing detected an alien attitude from [the solicitor] ...when he said that he was coming back to Ireland for good"; related that he was initially "afraid to ask" him "a question"; and wrote of the solicitor's reaction to me concerning his disclosed reply to the independent solicitor involved: "a cornered rat". The "rat", while a judge of the District Court, concerning what my father supposedly "felt":

> "Mr. [William] Ewing demurred strongly. He felt that Mr. M...y [another independent solicitor] acted for a number of local tenants who, he felt, were or might be pressing for Land Commission acquisition, in particular one local man who had been troublesome both to Mr. Ewing and to the Lennons. He did not want the Land Commission to become too interested in the land and what he was doing and was particularly anxious that it be unnecessary that any application for [Land Commission] consent either to leasing or sub-division be submitted."

Cornering the harasser: "Robert Ewing is raising cane"; and also his "rat": "Mr. Ewing knew exactly what he was doing" (lie such as: "knew exactly what he had borrowed"; and both lied that "Ewing kept visiting", rather than had returned "to Ireland for good"). And my father related how the harasser too generated anxiety concerning the Land Commission:

> "It would appear from my conversations with K...y that my neighbours were very interested in the possibility of the lands which I had inherited being taken over by the Land Commission and divided amongst them. He made it appear to me that his friendship with me would

help prevent any possibility of this happening." /"he was afraid they would put me wise to what he was doing."

The relevant logic therefore was that they alleged that my father and his local community were errant, "except to express the view" that one local man "has behaved totally honourably throughout the entire" locality, as had "the writer" of course:

> "We would point out [to the independent solicitor involved] that Mr. Ewing is not an old gentleman retreating into the armchair but is a robust middle aged man of around the 40 [closer to sixty than fifty] years of age..."

And "note the way the matter is twisted ...so as to make me appear the villain of the piece": "his son Robert is 20 years of age..."; and note my italics: "Robert is 20 years of age *and* Mr. Ewing reserves for himself the right to make such disposal of his property as may seem right to him at the time taking into account of course Roberts position *and* Mr. Ewing *and* the rest of family situation." Indeed: "*and* if there is to be a settlement of the [dwelling] property ...there will have to be an examination of the financial situation" /"*and* there would be divided interests" /"*and* if everybody who thought that they had a grievance either against the solicitor or the client were to behave in this fashion, a solicitors office would be a permanent battle ground." /"I have not been an obstacle ...*and* I resent his implication that I was such" /"Mr. Robert Ewing, who I attempted to assist by writing to his father [for example: "his anxieties"] to depict his [the vendor's] state of mind, [earlier version: "*and* subsequent visits *and* to try *and* assist in defusing family resentments I wrote to

Mr. Bill Ewing"] did in fact, threaten me with violence *and* threw books *and* papers both at me *and* on the floor. [earlier version: "he physically threatened me, threw my books *and* papers about the floor" /"he rushed from the office roaring *and* shouting *and* banging doors"] The suggestion of a polite exchange regarding his fathers age does not appear true to me *and* he most certainly *both* on that occasion *and* earlier ["earlier" threatening the solicitors with the State] had uttered threats regarding what he would do to his father, [contemporary lie: "threatening the writer *and* we may say yourself"] if he did not comply" /"*and* he was anxious" /"Mr. K...y has behaved totally honourably throughout ...at some considerable expense *and* trouble to himself" /"*and* Mr. K...y was certainly on the face of it a somewhat reluctant and concerned person who was worried..." /"in particular one local man who had been troublesome *both* to Mr. Ewing *and* to the Lennons. He did not want the Land Commission to become too interested in the land *and* what he was doing *and* was particularly anxious..." /"He decided to postpone discussions *and* would not go ahead with that proposed transaction" /"Mr. K...y would see his bank ...*and* Mr. Ewing took the map..." /"he had already drawn some £19,000 from ...K...y *and* ...K...y was pressed, apparently, in regard to the money." /"I deeply resent the statement that I deliberately *and* for profit unscrupulously assisted Mr. ...K...y ...I, at the time regarded Mr. Ewing as a friend *and* I was anxious to help him *and* dissuade him from using the lands as a milk cow for cash rather than a small and useful farm" /"Mr. Ewing appeared to have no interest [in farming] ... *and* proceeded against advice to make continued demands for loans and cash subventions." /"I attended to give evidence not for one or other party, ["interrupting, being technical, talking at length, breaking Mr. Ewing's train of thought, made it very difficult for Mr. Ewing to pin him down to any one point" during cross-examination] but as available to *both*." /"*and* he ["the surviving spouse"] is agreeable I think to accept this".

His son: "*and* I wrote back [concerning the allegations: "*and* damage he has caused to the property *and* threats he has made concerning same"] noting…"

The new solicitor: "*and* complicated" /"*and* dismissed each" /"*and* by …representing themselves." And "notes" of the harasser's evidence at the re-hearing: "*and* that my Solicitor would clarify this…" /"his Solicitor *and* friend" (senior counsel stating: "initially acting for …Ewing, *and* a friend of his") /"very well acquainted [first hearing: "I never had a better friend"] *and* even friendly" - "Ewing often said to me that I was his bank *and* that I need not fear lending money to him as I was buying land by doing so."

The third solicitors stated that the consent application had: "various inaccuracies", rather than state: 'lies'; and related: "may very well" and "quite likely", as: "might" ("in order to protect" the judge of the District Court); and specifically lied in order "to make me appear the villain of the piece":

> "Mr Robert Ewing [the only specific reference to the second co-defendant] is a son of Mr William Ewing *and* has been involved in some fracas on *and* around the land with Mr K…y. We [reference also to the future bar association president] have made it extremely clear to our clients as to the difficulties which they are facing…" [co-defendant Robert Ewing would advise St Brendan's church: "I am almost certain that we are facing what

an American would call 'a one trick pony'."] /"R...y &
C...y [the new solicitors involved since the future judge
of the District Court lied: "we will have to inform Mr.
...K...y of the contents thereof *and* let him take advice
on what action he wishes to take in respect of same"]
when they took over the matter [would obtain the Land
Certificate behind the vendor's back and support the
harasser's proposal to acquire most of the lawn] appear
to have made every attempt to transfer the part of the
property comprising the house and six acres back to Mr
Ewing [disregarding that the proposed application to the
Land Commission was a result of the dispute:] *and* they
sent an application form re Land Commission Consent
[involving lie that the re-transfer obligation was "a
verbal agreement"; and lie: "already had a legal right-
of-way" /"Consent apparently issued" despite no vendor
involvement, as he noted: "Robert Ewing blamed for
rift" - "accused wrongly"] to Mr Ewing for signature by
him"

My pleading: "and had attempted to force the Plaintiff's father
into a settlement on the eve of the hearing by representing that
his barrister was not available [note "and":] and that £2,000 was
immediately required from him to pay for a replacement." The
first Supreme Court (while not a quotation): "and attempted to
force the Plaintiff's father into a settlement on the eve of the
hearing by representing that his barrister was not available." /"*and*
it is his belief and understanding that there is a constitutional
obligation on this Court *and* that there was a constitutional
obligation on the Circuit Court (*and* the High Court on appeal

from it) to investigate those suspicions." /"his judgment was confined to a consideration of technical issues ..."rather than with any evaluation of the matters which are clearly of concern to the Plaintiff *and* are the subject of his complaint ...in these Courts"." /"However, Mr Ewing has said that he appreciates, *and* I can well understand that he would appreciate, the basic principle." /"Mr Ewing has reviewed the matter, he has pointed out that this appeal was, in his submission, necessary to obtain certainty. He expressed his appreciation for the judgment of this Court because it did as he said provide certainty *and* ["*and* he is agreeable I think to accept this"] finality in the matter."

And the word "or" was also "twisted": "a grievance either against the solicitor ["a typing error"] *or* the client" ("*and* we may say..."). The first Supreme Court: "The allegation that this firm of solicitors attempted [the fourth solicitors: "to set up the plaintiff *or* his father or attempted to force..."] *or* succeeded to..." The second Court: "allegations of negligence and fraud against the Law Society and a number of solicitors firms, who, at different times, had acted for (*or* against) the family." /"the matter of Abbeyville House *and* [note "his alleged":] his alleged unlawful imprisonment therein"; "his case as pleaded": [note "or to ...his character": "all issues that presently relate to either the plaintiff's enjoyment of his home (Abbeyville House), or to a public appreciation of his character as the present occupant of Abbeyville House, and..."] "all issues that presently relate to either the plaintiff's enjoyment of his home (Abbeyville House), and..." - "and [or to] his alleged ...imprisonment therein."

Thus whilst litigation begun by any lawyer states the word "and" between the parties, litigation begun by a lay-litigant effectively states "or"; the defendant is the legal profession:

"I gave a lift to Robert Ewing not knowing initially who he was. ["He willingly gave up a Saturday morning", "& has worked for me in his holidays from college"] As a result of that *and* subsequent visits ["much of it a result of his enthusiasm and endeavour"] ...I wrote to Mr. Bill Ewing setting out Robert's 'case'. This ...led to nothing *and* Robert Ewing instructed Mr. M...n solicitor to write to ["Bill" - as the same solicitor would relate to] me."

Thus would the judge of the District Court not relate that my father authorised the consultation, just as the said "solicitor" (the independent solicitor involved) would state the words: "strongly" and "anxious", and would not relate that my father had no independent legal advice.

The fourth solicitors neither invited me to meetings nor hearings: "the legal team did not seem to want my son by my side, and indeed I was warned, that the other side was making something of the fact that Robert was involved." "Can you find out if these people intend this matter ever to go back into court!!?"

Just as he thus asked St Brendan's church, I would ensure that he would "find out if" "the legal team" would perform, by not attending the re-hearing. I advised him: "It cannot be both it appears"; and co-defendant senior counsel would claim at the re-hearing, contrary to our notes and correspondence, that he was only representing the first co-defendant - as if the co-defendants were at loggerheads with one-another. Only I had also written of that senior counsel that he would refer to me at hearing as if I was "a dunce", the dictionary definition of which is: "Loggerhead; a blockhead: a dunce".

The first Supreme Court, addressing its 'dunce', claimed that the negligence panel solicitors had not been given "an opportunity" to defend the co-defendants; and the second Court lied that "the opportunity of reading documents beforehand ensures that no injustice is done to a litigant in person", and that my appeal involved a reference to costs (the litigation involved reference to costs, and such would be quoted by the Court). The routine being the question as to how ordered costs could be paid; not question as to whether or not hearing had been denied by lawyers, and by way of lies to both client/s and judge. The first Court: "On that basis it is clear that the claim against Mr K…y in the existing proceedings was rightly dismissed."

One local man particularly, and others; but subsequently neither caused anxiety; threat only from "this young man" - "aggressive Robert Ewing"? The judge of the District Court:

> "I asked him to remain while I called the Gardai but he rushed from the office" /"he expressed threats against his father if he did not immediately comply with his wishes [otherwise: "with his desires"] – he physically threatened me" /"he was anxious that immediate action be taken to assure the lands" [as the solicitor: "he seemed to think we were responsible"]

Rather: "we were responsible", and "I asked him to remain" for the blame-game, "but he rushed from the office…" "Robert [aged fourteen: "has a mature and enthusiastic approach to his work which has produced some excellent results"] …is a mature and conscientious boy who well deserves his success. Robert's attitude towards his work is sensible and positive" /"Again [just prior to first meeting the harasser] a very thoughtful and conscientious half-year's work with pleasing results." My initiatives were to remedy the isolation begun by the solicitor, not worsen it by inviting adverse report to any solicitor who might have engaged:

> "We [the independent solicitors involved] have been consulted by your son, Robert, who has expressed anxiety ...We know that your own Solicitor ...wrote to you ...and there is no need for us to repeat what has been stated..." /"Suffice it to say that Robert feels so strongly about the preservation of what is left of the estate that he decided to consult an independent solicitor and hence this letter." /"Robert feels very strongly that something will have to be done in the very near future ...and is, obviously, willing and anxious about the matter"

"In reality the 2" solicitors were "the same"?

The High Court: "Mr. [Robert] Ewing's view is strongly held." And second and first Supreme Court was "the same":

> "He [the harasser] alleged the Ewings were trespassing on the disputed lands [the land] and had obstructed a right of way to which he, [neither as "his neighbour" nor] as purchaser, claimed to be entitled."

> "The material prepared by Mr [Robert] Ewing is directed almost exclusively to [relating the discontinuity between the first hearing and re-hearing, and also the evidence supportive of the co-defendant pleading at the first] ...

the sale of the lands"/"almost exclusively [not] concerned
with the issue of land ownership."

The second Court lied: "He now says his concern …was not
really about the land" ("his father sold land"), and lied that I
claimed that the first Court quoted me, not 'misquoted' me; the
first Court indisputably 'misquoted' written pleadings:

> "a [the] trust" (purposeful misquotation of allegation
> concerning William Ewing's involvement with the
> solicitor and harasser, both "Roman Catholic") /"his
> [family's connection] father's connections" /"the conduct
> of ["the conduct of the Gardai and legal profession, set
> against the back-drop of the correspondence …between
> Taoiseach …and" co-defendant Robert Ewing] the Gardai
> and legal profession…may suggest a determination on
> the part of [the] Irish people themselves" /"his English
> references described [describe] him…"

"The official response" was that "the Court had had the
opportunity of reading the papers prior to the hearing".

And the case-law quoted (or purposely misquoted) by the
Court was relevant only to the harasser and his false "special
summons" (attached to exterior house doors as attempt to
generate anxiety again that the dwelling could be acquired;
in other words: "threatened by R…y, take the consequences if
not willing to settle"): "harassment and oppression", by way of
"proceedings brought for purposes other than the assertion of
legitimate rights" (the Court concluding thereby: "The action
is brought for an improper purpose, and not for the assertion of
legitimate rights").

The High Court had accepted the false summons (as would the third Supreme Court, despite no professional summons server's signature); disregarded my affidavits and evidence; and lied that the evidence was that the re-transfer obligation was "verbal" (indisputably "verbal" was a lie); the Court was thus example of how our involvement with the legal profession generally meant that we had less, not more, control of our rights ("I, therefore, left the meeting, in protest…" /"the *legal profession!!?*"). Village: "they treat people who disagree with them as if they were not just not equal to them but valueless"?[1] I advised him during "the delaying tactics": "It is the legal profession or Robert Ewing. It cannot be both it appears." And the High Court would deny me the right to insist that it choose between the original claim of the false "summons" (order for sale of the dwelling), and my reply – which involved anticipating that claim strategy; the Court adhered to the bully routine and ordered division of the dwelling by way of the routine lie, effectively: "The difficulties I see arising…"

Thus lawyers are generally not principally available to resolve misunderstanding or harassment, and are generally available to 'misunderstand' or harass. Just as judges do not clarify "best interest" or "best interests", rather lie; such as the first and second Supreme Court would lie by way of quoting my pleaded word "natural"; the denial of the legal system to my father naturally tended to generate a dispute, just as it had naturally tended to generate both immediate and file discovery, and the denial of the legal system to me subsequently inevitably led to proceedings against the State.

---

[1]   'Is equality a right?'

The negligence of the first Supreme Court meant that the State was entirely liable for the litigation involved, as it was not procedurally "fair" for me to again institute proceedings against the former Circuit Court plaintiff as would challenge the relevant orders obtained by him. The second Court did not allow costs against me as plaintiff against the State, as if to confuse relative to the liability for those proceedings, which the Court lied "was not possible to discern".

And thus the State had "further delayed and complicated" the dispute; just as it would further delay and complicate the legal issues until its disregard for the dispute could be finally imposed, irrespective of human rights: "a civil matter"; "harassment and oppression of other parties by multifarious proceedings"; "Robert Ewing blames one of his former solicitors"; "lawyers who have acted for or against"; "the plaintiff or his father or attempted"; "or succeeded"; "against the many lawyers engaged and involved"; "the plaintiff's point of view of those proceedings"; "Roberts point of view"; "is that the pressures of the litigation badly affected his father's health"; "Roberts case"; "to blame"; "a firm of solicitors"; "the case as pleaded"; "to pay the costs of unsuccessful proceedings"; "he did not think it would be fair"; "to pay the costs"; "I think he probably wants some concession"; "he seemed to think we were responsible".

My father wrote: "Was judge Cassidy responsible?" And recorded: "Robert Ewing spoke as a quiet intellectual, who ["contrary to what was being inferred by the other side"] had no bad feelings or aggressive nature." /"He was sad at what was taking place."

Neither the Law Society, [which had "steered" the vendor to negligence panel solicitors, and to choose between one of three such solicitors in its locality, rather than in his] nor the Land Commission, nor the Revenue Commissioners, while apparently cheated, had any interest in the fraud concerning them, rather simply deployed lawyers to obtain striking-out of the proceedings meant to relate their specific negligence which advantaged the litigation harassment.

Yet the judge of the District Court would vindicate my involvement: "He [William Ewing] told me that Mr. K…y owned what was precisely half of Abbeyville and might well own the whole lot [and] if things went well with himself that he might get the whole farm back. That certainly seemed impossible…" My father could not even get his dwelling back, just as he could not get back to the first hearing.

And the future bar association president also vindicated my involvement, by way of referring to my father's trust in the harasser, as follows: "As a result of this friendship Mr. K…y has taken advantage of Mr. Ewing." The harasser, concerning my father and the solicitor: "his solicitor and friend"; and to my father: "I have no friends in town."

A retired judge related his routine question to himself in court: "Who is exaggerating the most?" And such is the culture of the legal system, as devised by way of economic restriction to both State and litigant; and its component culture is therefore of being 'economical with the truth' – telling the truth is not considered helpful or clever, and reference to money is, irrespective of the truth. Thus while the fourth solicitors stated the word "scandalous" to me, they did not inform my co-defendant that judge Cassidy had ordered the plaintiff's motion costs (motions meant as "delaying tactics" and means to create debt) paid prior to any further hearing; thus re-hearing began as would most "suit the future Defendants". Just as co-defendant senior counsel was "banging the table", rather than provide pre-court preparation meeting; discovery effectively denied my attending meetings; and the High Court would claim to be concerned with technical issues (in order to deny hearing of the first proceedings alleging denial of hearings):

> "My only concern is ...to reach conclusions on the relatively technical questions ...I am confined to a consideration of technical issues ["application such as the present one is dealt with at a technical level"] ... rather than with any evaluation of the matters which are clearly of concern to the Plaintiff and are the subject of his complaint, but which are..."

The solicitor to my father prior to the involvement of any other solicitors: "my only desire [more personal than stating: 'my only concern', and he altered "faithfully" to "sincerely"] is to act for the benefit of yourself more than anybody else ["Written ...only because of Robert's alarm!"] ...you are ["One now knows that Mr. K...y was registered as owner at this point in time!"] the owner of the property".

"Indeed you are" the prime minister, wrote writers Antony Jay and Jonathan Lynn; "you are the owner"; note my italics:

> "In a case like this particular matter it is usually possible to come to some arrangement as between the surviving spouse *and* in this case the principal beneficiary yourself who in this case *you are* also being a co executor."

And also to be culturally "helpful", at least concerning "this particular matter", the first Supreme Court, having accepted neither allegation nor evidence from me, lectured as the minister for justice had about the legal system:

> "Mr Robert Ewing may be mistaken as to the manner in which courts of law seek to attain justice. In Ireland the Judicial system is adversarial. Each party asserts the legal rights claimed by him and puts forward the evidence available …the Judges to adjudicate upon the evidence and argument placed before them." /"The reference by Mr Robert Ewing to the decision ["of this Court in …1971"] …shows how misunderstandings may arise in relation to our judicial system."

Thus the State is involved in the "theft" of the lands that I had reported to the government, and that the third solicitors stated as the vendor alleging "no control".

And thus whilst State inquiry would conclude that my claim against the State was procedurally inevitable, and that the dispute concerned denial of the technical legal issues which would safeguard against the harasser dominating the dwelling, the second Supreme Court lied that I, not the purchaser, "wanted to deny" consequence of the vendor's signatures; just as the first Court lied concerning the Circuit Court litigation: "the proceedings concerning the land", and would not refer to the various money claims by which division of the dwelling would be ordered (if not obtained by way of 'negotiation'), irrespective of pleading.

In other words, the words "strongly" and "anxious" had "the same" origin as the "2" proceedings they were stated by the judge of the District Court to support; the "whole affair" would be "twisted" by the ethos that legal clients "cannot tell their own interests – that they should have the leave of the office before they do anything". I could tell our interests, and politely threatened his firm (while concluding a consultation with his son) with the State, just as judge Cassidy had reacted against "the document" and the son's nervousness:

> "You asked Mr. Ewing for signatures for money that you knew he did not receive? You knew he did not receive that money? *Didn't you? Didn't you?*"

The son's reaction to the dispute involved written lie: "this would not appear to be possible from the documentation we hold in our office"; the impossible was to "forward you Land Certificate" which he no-longer possessed.

I wrote to my co-defendant: "I was thinking about what you have said, and what …k [the negligence panel solicitor] …has said to me in the more recent past, and it is interesting what you said to me over the phone regarding [him] …using me [at some future time, which he did: "We have made it extremely clear"] as an excuse to change direction." That solicitor would lie to him; and note my italics:

> "It appears now that due to the delay in the Galway proceedings coming on for trial *you are* now changing your instructions *and* wish to proceed with an action ["for professional negligence"] …before the outcome of the Galway proceedings is known."

Only I had reported this third solicitors to the government as: "not taking any notice of my father's wishes", such as this correspondence proves; this solicitor, prior to my report:

> "I confirm that as soon as I receive the [judge's and his son's] Statement[s] I will consider the contents of same [he subsequently received them but would not notify that he had until accepting dismissal] and forward copies to Counsel and yourself *and* at that time to make a final decision as to the question of going ahead with a professional negligence action"

His dismissal correspondence contradicts that he wrote any letter concerning the Statement/s, and contradicts, thus:

> "In light of the fact that you no longer wish us to act on your behalf in the manner originally agreed I am reluctant to continue acting on your behalf in any capacity." /"When I received instructions from you initially [lie such as: "when they took over the matter"] ...it was clearly understood *and* agreed by you..." /"It was always the view of ourselves and Counsel that it was vital to await the outcome of the Galway proceedings. You and I have had numerous meetings and telephone conversations in relation to the matter *and* you have never been in any doubt as to my advice and Counsel's advice in this regard."

"You know very well"; the fourth solicitors remarked: "scandalous", to me, having sought the discovery order as means to rely on routines to exclude my involvement ("the solicitor in question never intended my son Robert to be involved in case proceedings, something I felt from a very early stage but could not fathom or understand"), knowing that the first hearing was obtained by way of my initiatives (strategies to obtain the necessary adversarial relations). My co-defendant "pressured" that solicitor to obtain hearing date (hearing with judge Cassidy relative to the three-day hearing which he had not finalised), and co-defendant senior counsel ensured averting that hearing by way of meeting at which he would lie that the plaintiff had "lost" his senior counsel. My co-defendant was subsequently "assured" of second meeting "well before the hearing date", but it was delayed until the hearing was imminent (as had been attempted by junior counsel with the second solicitors in October, 1988, until I intervened), just as he had alleged: "delaying tactics of the legal profession". Hearing was thus obtained after a number of tactical motions and judge Cassidy's death.

"The modern rules have a distinguished ancestry", states textbook foreword by a judge of the Supreme Court, only that was no-longer true:

> "In my view the learned [High Court] Judge was entirely correct as a matter of law and commendably sensitive in explaining his functions in that way."

And the minister had been "entirely correct as a matter of law and commendably sensitive"? He could have intervened against the judge of the District Court; but both the minister and the legal profession routinely oppose litigation against components, and accept litigation against the public: "matters at issue can be dealt with by the Courts"; the State can say "seem" and change it to "deem", rather than accept anything from the public, vilified as the element inclined to think that money should dictate; just as the harasser lied: "Ewing asked …for …the first loan" (and his senior counsel had the same tune: "asked …K…y for loans"), and such lie received no reply, except at the first hearing.

"It is necessary to understand", states legal textbook; and the supposedly "commendably sensitive" judgment thus referred to the rule term: "scandalous", since it was contrary to the "delicately" and "understanding" lie routine, and not least because it was quoted by such defendant as had already scandalously denied hearings; the judgment therefore began with explanation as to "its context in the Rule book". Thus "excuse" to refer to technical issues had routinely been deployed; "the Courts" would not process the inconvenient case, and therefore would conclude that the law was "expressly" at variance with "the plaintiff's point of view" (which none of the legal professionals involved would relate as the co-defendant appeal having failed on account of the mistreatment of the co-defendants between the order for discovery and the first possible appeal hearing). The second Supreme Court: "By this time [reference to the appeal from the re-hearing] William Ewing [who had represented himself throughout the three-day hearing, until the judge advised him to engage solicitors] was representing himself." "He [Robert Ewing] held the State culpable." "He also sought to involve the European Court of Human Rights". Thus would the Court not relate that the Disciplinary Tribunal of the High Court had been involved; just as the first Court would neither relate which solicitors were considered negligent nor whether or not such application was considered subsequent to the Circuit Court litigation, and nor whether or not any application occurred.

Thus both solicitors and judges exploited procedural routines, rather than relate that the legal profession caused the dispute and would not resolve it; as my father related concerning the unpaid motion costs: "solicitors fault – not telling me"; only "telling" is routinely not being told: "Both the common law and public policy dictate there must be finality in proceedings between parties" /"There must come a point when there is finality in litigation."

"It is necessary to understand", therefore, that while such legal professionals claim that legal textbooks tell practically everything, such books tell practically nothing; it is evidence that tells us practically everything:

> "Primarily he [William Ewing, while contesting the debt order obtained by way of exploiting the change-over of solicitors] wishes me [the third solicitors] to hold it [funds equivalent to the pre-dispute debt claimed by the harasser] so that …I can off my own bat inform the Judge or the Solicitors for the other side that the money is actually in my possession."

"It is necessary to understand" that my co-defendant would rather understand the textbook, and that commonly there is pre-occupation with money: "letters [from the independent solicitor involved] which [did not] accuse Mr. K…y of deliberately setting out to take possession of the property for little payment. Mr. K…y has behaved totally honourably throughout" /"himself produced a notebook recording the moneys he had lent to Mr. Ewing [the monies claimed paid for the land obviously involved rent payment, rather than produced the sale sum] together with evidence of lodgment of moneys to Mr. Ewing's bank account" (stated the fourth solicitors, irrelevantly); just as the first Supreme Court lied that the legal profession held file evidence advantageous to the fourth solicitors:

> "That contention appears to be at variance with the facts as they appear from the order of the High Court. The allegation …is not supported by any evidence."

And just as the co-defendant senior counsel referred to "the document" sums, the second Court lied: "The pleadings evince Mr. [Robert] Ewing's concern regarding a number of perceived irregularities"; the Court would not relate that the sale involved one solicitor only (thus to lecture: "our judicial system", and thereby conclude: "must now be understood"); not relate that the purchaser was obligated to re-transfer the dwelling (and had not done so); and not relate that the co-defendants allegedly had not been heard (pleaded to the second Court as: "The Circuit Court heard what was supposed to suit the future Defendants…"). And since the allegation: "to suit the future Defendants" could not be stated as "now says", the Court would continue not to refer to it, thereby maintaining appearance of straightforward costs order issues – a straightforwardness such as the solicitor began by denying my father the adversarial system:

> "he has substantially paid the greater part of the purchase money…" /"if there is to be a settlement …there will have to be an examination of the financial situation over all in relation to these lands"

And "Little Ship Street" responded to the litigation against the State by lie that the proceedings principally concerned money, and were "proceedings to be had" (meant as reference to An Garda Síochána). "This appears to be a civil matter"? "Mr. Robert Ewing", "who is anxious to have certain property restored in the family name", lied the minister for justice. "Mr. Robert Ewing, who I attempted to assist by writing..."

I responded to the first Circuit Court summons to me by comment on it: "Bullshiter"; only every legal professional who was or would become involved had the same routine: "government is about not answering";[1] effectively: "Of course Mr. Robert Ewing has no interest in the lands and has no right to make any of the statements or anything else that have been made by him."

To whom are we listening?

"P.S Please provide instructions in separate letter from any other comment you wish to make."

I advised my co-defendant prior to co-defendant senior counsel "banging the table", quoting the Duke of Wellington at Waterloo thus: "Hard pounding this, gentlemen; we shall see who can pound the hardest."

"The case against" the official thus "determined once and for all"; senior counsel at the Four Courts "banging the table"; and senior judge at the Four Courts concluding: "that point has now arrived"; individuals not to be acknowledged as understanding law can never arrive at "that point" where "it must now be understood", just as individuals not permitted to enter the Law Library are not permitted to it - whether they understand that rule or not.

---

[1]   Writers Jay and Lynn

Indeed, the legal "profession generally only has one case – every case is treated the same": "instructions ...separate" /"separately issued".

And, indeed, irrespective of instructions and proceedings "every word they use is convenient to them." "Mr. Ewing wanted further very substantial funds" /"he wanted the funds and was prepared *and* wished ...for sale." /"*and* Mr. Ewing was not prepared to wait for additional monies" /"Mr. Ewing was not prepared to wait for the issue of [Land Commission] consent before receiving funds. It was obvious to me..."

Any other observations?

It was obvious to me that my father wanted a solicitor. The Supreme Court: "William Ewing was advised by a firm of solicitors in the area" ["I asked him to remain ...but he rushed from the office"] /"This [second] firm was later replaced by a second firm of solicitors" ["Mr. Ewing was not prepared to wait"] /"Then there was a further change of solicitor" ["Mr. Ewing was not prepared to wait"] /"This is a helpful summary which ...for all judges of the superior courts, will be statements of the obvious." "Of course ...Mr. K...y has behaved totally honourably throughout..."

"And when the Czechs were beaten-up trying to combat his [Henlien's] fifth columnists, [generally only "harassment and oppression"] Hitler ["never interested in legitimate ambitions"[1]] screamed the Germans were being persecuted, and threatened ["it must now be"] war..."[2]

---

[1]   Ivone Kirkpatrick (1959)

[2]   USA service information film 2

Market forces

"It would be a dangerous illusion to think that, if
war once starts, it will come to an early end even if
a success on any one of the several fronts on which
it will be engaged should have been secured."
Neville Chamberlain to Hitler, August 1939

Churchill had one ear for history and the other for politics, and certainly listened to Chamberlain, who said long before he said it: "we will never surrender" (March 1939).

"Long before Munich he [Chamberlain] had shocked substantial sections of opinion by his frank and completely realist assessment of the strength and weakness of the League of Nations. When it was clear that members of the League, for good reasons or bad, were not prepared to involve themselves in war over questions in which they themselves had no direct interest, it was obviously idle to pretend that there was any such thing as 'collective security' on which nations could confidently rely for their own protection."[1]

"There was at this date no 'League of Nations', [a statement generated by reference to the United Nations] …and if ever there was a phrase without meaning it was 'collective security' as opposed to national security under the conditions of the later thirties."[2]

---

[1]   Edward Wood (1957)

[2]   D.C. Somervell (1950)

"The P.M. gave an impressive narrative of events in Austria, but wisely did not commit the country to anything but greater efforts." /"He said he had come clean round from Winston's idea of a Grand Alliance [an alliance of European powers with Russia] to a policy of diplomatic action and no fresh commitments."[1]

"In July [1938] Hitler sent a message to Chamberlain that, if Britain were to persuade Benes, the Czech President, to cede the Sudetenland, Germany would not attack Czechoslovakia."[2] "That was Chamberlainism"?

> "Hitler can make certain legitimate demands. So long as his demands fall …fairly and squarely on the old Wilsonian principle of nationality or self-determination."

"That was" not "old", but "an art of a highly experimental kind, probably in its infancy and proceeding by trial and error to ends which it is impossible to foresee";[3] as was this:

> "Everyone must recognise that the Prime Minister is pursuing a policy of a most decided character and of capital importance. He has his own strong view ["Mr. Ewing's view is strongly held…"] about what to do, and about what is going to happen. He has his own standard of values; he has his own angle of vision. ["I believe it is based on a misunderstanding…"] He believes ["that the conduct of the Defendants or, at least some of them, was to say the least, suspect, and it is his belief and understanding…"] that he can make a good settlement

---

[1] Geoffrey Dawson, March 1938

[2] Roy Denham (1996)

[3] J.A. Spender (1938)

for Europe and for the British Empire by coming to terms with Herr Hitler and Signor Mussolini ["Robert is …anxious about the matter, he …feels very strongly that something will have to be done in the very near future"] …and we are going to learn, in a comparatively short time, what he proposes should happen to us.

The Prime Minister is persuaded that Herr Hitler seeks no further territorial expansion upon the Continent of Europe…"[1]

"That was" Churchillism; only the "Grand Alliance" was not entirely his "idea":

"In face of such problems, to be badgered and pressed to come out and give a clear, decided, bold, and unmistakable lead, show 'ordinary courage', and all the rest of the twaddle, is calculated to vex the man who has to take the responsibility for the consequences. As a matter of fact, the plan of the 'Grand Alliance', as Winston calls it, had occurred to me long before he mentioned it…"

And as for "the show ship" initialing "I.K." or "I.K.B.":

"U.S.A. and U.K. in combination represent a force so overwhelming that the mere hint of the possibility of its use is sufficient to make the most powerful of dictators pause …the trouble is that public opinion in a good part of the States still believes it possible for America to stand outside Europe and watch it disintegrate, without being

---

[1]   Winston Churchill, subsequent to the Munich agreement debate

materially affected herself …she cannot be depended on for help if we should get into trouble."

"That was Chamberlainism": "Germany would not attack Czechoslovakia" if Hitler feared the result; "it must be admitted that in 1937 it was becoming rather late in the day to do the only effective thing, namely, to knock Hitler on the head."[1]

"There is good evidence that orders for the invasion on the 25th August [1939] were actually given and then cancelled at the last moment because H. wavered."

Certainly, 'the house that Hitler built' was "not built up to the strengths to which he was entitled" by "an Anglo-German agreement, which he continually declared to be his greatest ambition". He would rather appease than provoke the "top dog of Europe", "since it forms a vast community of language and culture together with the U.S.A." and "has always [such was his thesis and agenda] …to carry through to victory any struggle that it once enters upon, no matter how long such a struggle may last or however great the sacrifice that may be necessary or whatever the means that have to be employed; and all this even though the actual military equipment at hand may be utterly inadequate when compared with that of other nations." "Never from No. 10 did any order come to slow up anything", remarked the former pilot and parliamentarian, Harold Balfour:

> "I saw him wave that piece of paper and read the declaration that he and Hitler had that day signed, resolving to settle peacefully all future differences between our two countries. Why he said what he did I

---

[1]   Ivone Kirkpatrick (1959)

shall never know. [reference to the *subsequent* speech that day, stating "peace with honour" and also "peace for our time" at "No. 10"] Did he believe it? Was it emotional fatigue and reaction in a man of advancing years who had flown half across Europe in air travel conditions very different than those of today? Did he believe the words "peace with honour"? Did he regret and distrust almost at once? All this will never be answered with certainty. What I do know is that none of this can be reconciled with the urgent drive ["over the next twelve months to prepare the R.A.F. for war and to build up quick expansion of our aircraft industry. Never from No. 10 did any order come to slow up anything. On the contrary, we were encouraged and supported to double our efforts"] ...in the year left to us and for the air, I repeat, 'Thank God for Munich'."

Ambassador Nevile Henderson, on the other hand, advised against "a man of advancing years":

> "I believe that, if we are not too niggardly, Germany will keep her word, at any rate for a foreseeable period. One cannot legislate for more. And particularly so, if we take it for granted that she *will* keep her word. The surest way of getting her to break it is to doubt. That is elementary."

He advised Chamberlain to "go as far as he possibly can" toward accepting Hitler's claims, "even if we don't like it". And indisputably, Chamberlain's initial speech on his return from Munich was as staged as any of his presentations to the newsreels:

"If he [Hitler] signs it [the anglo-german declaration] and sticks to it that will be fine, but if he breaks it that will convince the Americans of the kind of man he is. I [Chamberlain] will give the maximum publicity to it when I return to London."

Clement Attlee would learn of him: "Very able and crafty."

"My impression is that Chamberlain has the country behind him on this issue of peace or war", noted Bruce Lockhart ("a sound and independent journalist", "half-way between the career diplomatist and the individual expert"). That was elementary, irrespective of whether or not Hitler would be deterred; and Chamberlain "would help to educate American public opinion to act more with us".

However, Lockhart, as unaware that Chamberlain's task to lead public opinion had a measure of consideration for "the educative power of events" (a particularly necessary measure concerning the United States, as "the isolationists there are so strong and so vocal"), wanted more certainty as to "the armament which she needed", and whether or not the persuading would deter Japan or plan (or plant) more (or less) "Cherry trees":

April 1938 (diary): "Saw [the foreign affairs under-secretary] Van [Vansittart] who talked to me very freely about situation. He has no use for Nevile Henderson whom he regards as greatest menace."

October 1938 (diary): "Harold Nicolson speaking yesterday attacked Chamberlain for neglecting the advice of his experts like Van who was consistently right and listening to Sir Horace Wilson 'whose advice was never inconvenient'." /"Rex [Leeper] also told me ["Chamberlain today does his own foreign policy (with Horace Wilson), and Foreign Office have a tag: 'If at first you can't concede, fly, fly, fly again.'"] that he had tried very hard to persuade the Government to appoint me as assistant to [Walter] Runciman when latter was sent on his mission to Czechoslovakia. Decided, however, that it would be too dangerous, as I knew too much! In other words, Germans would object to me as biased in favour of Czechs!"

October 1947: "His [Chamberlain's] own speeches, too, lacked force, ["and nothing could have been more pathetic than his quotation of: 'If at first you don't succeed, try, try, try again'."] …ninety-nine per cent. of the American correspondents were on the side of the democracies and against the dictators and performed a noble and notable task in awakening their own countrymen to the German danger."

Chamberlain "performed a noble and notable task"; "all strategies are abstractions which exist only in the minds of interested people … every strategy is an invention, a figment of someone's imagination".[1] "I sincerely believe", he wrote to the archbishop of Canterbury, "that we have at last opened the way to that general appeasement which alone can save the world from chaos." Only Churchill was disinclined to rule-out the past parliamentary allegation that "old Neville" regarded war "not as a possibility, but as a certainty":

"through cheering crowds …he said to Halifax …'all this will be over in three months'; but …he waved his

---

[1] Quinn, Mintzberg, James

piece of paper again and used these words …'I believe it
is peace for our time.'"

However, parliament had heard "all" that before:

> "I [Chamberlain] do not know why that conversation
> should give rise to suspicion, still less to criticism. I
> entered into no pact. I made no new commitments. There
> is no secret understanding. Our conversation ["that
> conversation" with Hitler which resulted in the signing
> of "that piece of paper"] was hostile to no other nation."

And Halifax would yet again take Churchill to task for "dead in
three months time":

> "Churchill did Chamberlain less than justice …that
> Chamberlain was concerned to mislead the public into
> the acceptance of a belief which he did not himself
> share" - "no one could fairly charge him with lack of
> frankness" - "he was concerned with the spirit in which
> he believed Hitler had signed the declaration, and which
> at that moment he was disposed to trust."

Yet Halifax knew that Henderson had advised a diplomatic trust,
and that Chamberlain had encouraged ministers to trust during
the crisis by declaring that he believed Hitler respected their
immediate consultative agreements; ultimately stating: "he could
be relied upon unless something quite unexpected occurred",
even "would be better rather than worse than his word". Thus,
whilst Hitler initially gave Chamberlain "the impression that
here was a man who could be relied upon when he had given

his word", and whilst Chamberlain had replied: "this time it is different; this time he has made his promises to me",[1] Halifax was prepared to leave the controversy where it began: "one person at least is completely satisfied that you are doing the right thing – no matter what the result."[2] As concerned immediate result, the goodwill of the German people and Hitler's accepting responses had encouraged Chamberlain's hopes, not as to whether or not postponing intervention was "the right thing", but as concerned averting the necessity for war.

Another historian concluded, however, that History "could fairly charge" Chamberlain with 'shamrock rearmament tea', even irrespective of St Patrick's Day:

> "'*What reliance*,' he cried bitterly in a speech at Birmingham, '*can be placed upon any other assurances that come from the same source?*'"[3]

"I [Chamberlain] should like to say that he ...seems to me to be completely divorced from reality. He is a victim of phrases and words"; "a dictator made him instinctively doubt the permanence of any settlement"; only he could not "reverse the methods and habits of peace as long as there was a chance of Hitler keeping his word".[4] And yet he achieved "a much sounder guarantee than could possibly otherwise have been the case",[5] as appearing "a nice kind old gentleman, who would not ever want to treat Germans roughly and unfairly", only critics thought "a

---

[1]   Cited by Leonard Mosley
[2]   Eamon de Valera
[3]   Stephen King-Hall (1961)
[4]   Templewood (1954)
[5]   Australian parliament (1940)

business-man's outlook" sounder than being "threatened with an umbrella from spinsters (who want pensions in return)": "my critics have applauded, without apparently understanding". His critics would not be postponed:

> "We ["Mr. M...y"] certainly would want some kind of a Guarantee of some nature ...£1,000 and if we could see some light that the balance would be guaranteed, but we have a feeling Mr. [William] Ewing might just flit back to England and leave us with nothing, and we got that impression very clearly from his son."

And whilst another historian more respected his balance, gave more credit, and "could see some light": "the essential fact about his policy of appeasement is not that he accepted Hitler's word, but that he pursued his plans so stubbornly in spite of his distrust",[1] Chamberlain was accustomed to administrative fights, not flights, and would pursue his objective even in spite of his trust: "If he signs it..." /"if he breaks it..." Thus, at the height of the crisis, taxed tea-leaves were not dispersing: "he had reluctantly come to the conclusion that Hitler's profession of limited objectives was not sincere".[2] Clearly the trivialities were "for some of his enemies to propagate and their dupes to believe":[3]

> Bermingham ("St Patrick's Day", 1939): "as I am still sound in wind and limb, I hope that I may have a few more years before me in which to give what service I can to the State if that should be wanted."

---

[1]   W.N. Medlicott
[2]   26th September 1938
[3]   C.B. Pyper (1962)

Brummagem (television drama, 1981): "as he felt still sound in mind and limb, he hoped he might have a few more years before him in which to give what service he could to the State."[1]

He concluded to parliament:

"I cannot help feeling that if, after all, war had come upon us, the people of this country would have lost their spiritual faith altogether. As it turned out the other way, I think we have all seen something like a new spiritual revival, and I know that everywhere there is a strong desire among the people to record their readiness to serve..." - "I hope they will not read into those words ["peace for our time"] more than they were intended to convey."

As for "the spirit in which he believed Hitler had signed": their interpreter thought he had signed the declaration "with a certain reluctance". Yet if "Chamberlain's phrase gave too much credit to the word of Hitler",[2] he was "glad of it; I do not take Hitler's peace professions at their face value", "credit to the word of Hitler" was some kind of a guarantee for credit, rather than simply state: "we may yet secure peace for our time, but I never meant to suggest that we should do that ...unless the consciousness exists, not here alone, but elsewhere, that behind the diplomacy is the strength to give effect to it."

"Every one of my single conditions were met", explained Hitler, but Germany had not only been influenced by "a

---

[1]   Brideshead Revisited
[2]   Maugham (1954)

magnificent character"[1] ("terribly over-praised for having done
no more than was my clear and obvious duty"), propaganda had
been deployed by way of radio to convince the German people
that Chamberlain was intervening to avert the risking of another
"great war", just as radio was deployed to convince the British
people to accept whatever he advised (and deployed during
the war, most successfully, to maintain Cumberland turf - at
Montevideo):

> "How horrible, fantastic, incredible it is that we should be
> digging trenches and trying on gas-masks here because
> of a quarrel in a far-away country between people of
> whom we know nothing. ["nothing that France or we
> could do could possibly save Czechoslovakia from being
> overrun ...Russia is 100 miles away"] It seems still more
> impossible that a quarrel which has already been settled
> in principle should be the subject of war."

"I can't possibly let a man of his age come all this way; I must
go to London."

"No one really knew what was happening at that time."[2]
Only the guarantees to Poland, Roumania, Greece and Turkey
persuaded Douglas Reed that he, at least, had not been so "far-
away" in September 1938:

> "it's all a long way away in countries we know nothing
> about, [Czechoslovakia] we must guarantee those more
> distant countries which we know still less about."

---

[1]   Margot Asquith (1940)
[2]   Anthony Hopkins

"Over and over again Canning lays it down that you should never menace unless you are in a position to carry out your threats". Chamberlain, thus "fortified" prior to first flying to Germany not "to tell Hitler now that, if he used force, we should at once declare war", advised the public that "we cannot in all circumstances undertake to involve the whole British Empire in war simply on her [the Czech] account".

"He used one reference which will be interpreted in Germany as a justification of Ribbentrop's insistence that 'we will never fight for Czechoslovakia'. He said 'however much we may admire a gallant little country, it is a very serious thing to commit the people of the British Empire to fighting for it'."[1]

"Even in this country there would have been no unity behind it."[2] Chamberlain stated: "the whole British Empire in war", but no one had "a pretext" for international consent: "Vansittart never offered a fully coherent critique of the government's assumptions and actions."[3] Indeed, "no one, not even the most eminent of the critics, knew when or indeed if Germany would break Hitler's promises and begin a European war."[4] Yet television drama would remain deferential to Reed, and would again misquote the advice:

> "We don't intend to involve the whole British Empire in war simply because of a quarrel in a far away country between people of whom we know nothing"[5]

---

[1] Robert Bruce Lockhart diary
[2] Geoffrey Dawson (1940)
[3] Michael Newman (1978)
[4] Maugham (1954)
[5] The Remains of the Day (1993)

Eamon de Valera had written to him: "I believe you will be successful. Should you not be so, you will be blamed..."

"You need professionals to run your affairs, or you're heading for disaster."[1] Or heading for "Black Thursday" and a scramble, consequently, for Yugoslav credit? "What we do need is to be a sufficiently unattractive hedgehog", advised Warren Fisher. And as Stanley Baldwin remarked while prime minister: not concern as to non-return of lent matches ("The era of ...consequences") but war, had first call on Churchill, even if Halifax was unlikely to agree with him:

> "Perhaps the greatest difficulty in the conduct of foreign affairs, and the one least appreciated by those not actually engaged in it, is the fact that the ideal policy is scarcely ever practicable."

"Diplomacy is the art of saying 'Good doggie' while you are looking for a stick."[2] "One of the most tragic and ironic scenes in all history."[3] "You have only to look at the map", noted Chamberlain, understanding that diplomacy is not the art of "digging trenches and trying on gas-masks", even as digging "Hitler's capacity to put himself temporarily into quite different and even contradictory moods".[4] "Nearly every one of my critics make the mistake of over-simplifying the problems I have to face. What is more tiresome is that they assume I am doing the same thing. But I assure you I am not such a 'mug' as is generally

---

[1]   The Remains of the Day (1993)

[2]   Quoted as "Anonymous"

[3]   USA service information film 2

[4]   Sumner Welles (1940)

supposed!"[1] "The day may come when my much cursed visit to Munich will be *understood*."[2] "No greater tragedy has overtaken any Prime Minister in this century."[3] "He missed the bus" when he "promised us all peace forevermore"?[4]

> "It was then he ["Neville Chamberlain, the Prime Minister"] showed the kindly, human side so few saw, but those who did valued highly. He patted my shoulder, called me by my Christian name and said that he was only sorry that I [Balfour] had been left in this isolated position for so long."

"Is there general appeasement?" Churchill asked, concerning the Anglo-Italian agreement of April, 1938. "I can't tell you what a help Neville is to me. I don't know what I should do without him." "'Out of this nettle, danger, we pluck this flower, safety.'" Only Louis Bromfield thought the flower "a halo", as would anyone who would pat the shoulder of the careerist "power élite" of "Washington or Moscow":

> "You must be white in colour; male; wear collar and tie and a dark suit; and able to spend most of your life indoors sitting down. You must also be able to dictate reasonably grammatical English. Oratory – once highly regarded – is no longer required. Anyone capable of reading from typescript can go to the highest place. These are the bare essentials. The right parents are a considerable asset. It is

---

[1]   To H.A. Gynne, January 1940

[2]   Margot Asquith's recollection

[3]   Swinton (1966)

[4]   Narrator Michael Dean

still best to come from 'the nobility and gentry', though it is probably a mistake to be the eldest son of a peer. Parents from the professional class are good, particularly if they pay surtax. Rich business men, oddly, not at all good. If you are so foolish as to be born into the industrial working class, then you must get out of it by winning a scholarship to a grammar school or, failing this, by becoming either a trade union official or a WEA tutor. If you are born of an agricultural labourer, you should give up at the start. The right education helps. It is of little moment what you learn, though Latin is still probably the most useful subject and any form of science a handicap; the important thing is where you learn. Eton remains by far the best bet; Winchester runs it close in the Labour Party. Otherwise prefer a first-rate grammar school to a minor public school and run away to sea rather than to a secondary modern. Oxford and Cambridge are so obvious a requirement as hardly to need mention. Any other university can be valued only for the instruction it provides. As to accomplishments, it is no longer necessary to ride a horse, shoot, fish, or even play bridge. In fact, the less accomplished you are outside your work the better. And even at work it is wiser to seem devoted rather than clever."[1]

"This he [Chamberlain] could not understand at all. With great simplicity he said that he had only tried to do what was right." "He gave me no warning, he just sent for me …at the end of May 1938." "This decision cost the R.A.F. at least a thousand Spitfires which should have been in reserve when the Battle of Britain started."

[1]   A.J.P. Taylor (1957)

"But I don't think there should be much dispute":[1] "Chamberlain concentrated on what could be done in peacetime to deter Germany, and to avoid defeat at the outset of war if deterrence failed."[2] Meantime, there was to be no "signal" to Hitler to step up the armament race: "wars are won not only now with arms and men, they are won with the reserves of resources and credit"; yet the doctor concluded: "Chamberlain and Wilson still clung to appeasement" /"Even after Munich there was ...appeasement"?

"I have confidence in recommending this boy",[3] "I don't mean to go to sleep". Munich was a crisis, not a curriculum:

> "I [Chamberlain] believe the double policy of rearmament and better relations with Germany and Italy will carry us safely through the danger period, if only the Foreign Office will play up".

"From the first he was certain that the man was partially mad. He was equally sure that what Hitler said today, he might contradict tomorrow. None the less, he believed that he could be influenced, and that although his acts had been bad in the past, they might be better in the future."[4] Only many people would ultimately judge appeasement while "bedeviled by a confusion between 'was' and 'should have been' – between what actually happened and what observers think ought to have happened";[5] and consequently the least objective of his critics clung to media confusion as to "the glamour boys" and the aspirin which the

---

1   Swinton (1966)
2   G.C. Peden (1979)
3   Headmaster C.G. Shankey (1945)
4   Templewood (1954)
5   Christopher Hill

Italian ambassador thought had "broken the evil spell" ("you have been human, while unfortunately traditional diplomacy sometimes loses touch with humanity"):

> "The fact is that he [Chamberlain] has clung ["to appeasement"?] to office like a limpet, that his motive has been personal vanity, and that he has used his power to push forward his friends and toadies to the great detriment of the public interest. When the country and the House of Commons would finally have no more of him, he clung frantically ["to appeasement"?] to 10 Downing Street and had literally to be thrown-out, and in spite of all ["still clung to appeasement"?] is still in the War Cabinet."[1]

"I thought of government as a comparatively simple thing requiring only that those who took part in it should have a faculty for public speaking and the kind of intellectual distinction valued by universities, but now I thought of it as the most difficult and complicated of all the arts" – "an art of" appeasement. "He [William Ewing] is a boy of excellent character, and his conduct has always been very satisfactory." "I try to warn myself against the dangers that beset all Prime Ministers, who are apt to be told only the agreeable things". "Good man", telegrammed Roosevelt. And Churchill would have said the same:

> "I felt it right to apologise for my inept handling of the situation. I said that if he [Chamberlain] felt that he had lost personal confidence in me as well as my losing the government a precious day of Parliamentary time in a

---

[1]   Cecil King diary (1940)

congested session, I should have no course other than to offer him my resignation."[1]

"There are not many positive services which the historian can do for the State and in a wider sense for the world, higher than that of tracing the causes of wars".[2] "You need professionals ...for ... things you and I don't understand".

"Is this the end of an old adventure, or is it the beginning of a new?" "I take the same view as Winston, to who's excellent" speech the United States had "been listening":

> "...as Winston calls" /"there will be many, including Winston, who will say..."

Only "proper advisors"[3] considered themselves the "proper advisors", just as parliament considered itself the engineer:

> "the final long-drawn-out agonies that preceded the actual declaration of war were as nearly unendurable as could be. We [Chamberlain and co.] were anxious to bring things to a head ...and meantime the House of Commons was out of hand, torn with suspicions, and ready (some of them...) to believe the government guilty of any cowardice and treachery"

"He brought to international affairs a business-man's outlook; but he made the mistake of thinking that in Hitler and Mussolini

---

[1]   Harold Balfour (1973)

[2]   Cyril Falls (1946)

[3]   Robert Bruce Lockhart (1947)

he had men on whose word he could rely."[1] Rather, he was "one of the most misunderstood men of his time …for thinking he could 'deal with dictators'."[2] Or thinking he could rely on Roosevelt, "which some of my critics have applauded, without apparently understanding the connection between diplomatic and strategic strength which, nevertheless, has been always stressed by the wisest diplomats and statesmen of the past". His opinion of the revolutionary German regime prior to the Munich crisis: "utterly untrustworthy and dishonest". And such would be the blame-game lie that Poland had invaded Germany; that Poland had been handed a "blank cheque" for aggression; as if Chamberlain "might just flit back to England and leave" Hitler "one of the most misunderstood men of his time".

"The verdict of history will condemn the statesman who was unable to take the responsibility of a bold decision, and sacrificed the hopes of the future to the present need of peace."[3] "Unable" and "unable", or the whole appeasement controversy is that it was "a bold decision", and would decide (as Chamberlain had tabled), that "business-men make better rulers than lawyers"?

> "One of his great qualities indeed was the unflinching honesty of his mind which tended to make him shrink from any economy of unpalatable truth. No one had ever been a more devoted and passionate lover of freedom…"[4]

"I felt I was indispensable, for no one else could carry out my policy". The Italian ambassador: "I wish him every success." "I

---

[1]   I.M.M. MacPhail (1961)

[2]   C.B. Pyper (1962)

[3]   Friedrich Von Bernhardi (1914)

[4]   Edward Wood (1957)

wish him [Robert Ewing, aged fifteen] every success." /"A mature and extremely helpful member of the tutor group, always helpful both to members of staff and to other members of the group."

"Well, that's right";[1] the factory floor fought the dictator, and Chamberlain did, and he and the factory floor, rather than the theorists versus the blame-game phenomenon, won.

In other words, "long before" the dictator began "banging the table", I had begun a verdict of history favourable to "the central brain"; a project not blaming any competent administrator, but educating the inept, like Reed, who blamed him and would, thereby, trouble social order to achieve an administrative excellence already obtained. The blame-game had twice targeted a competent administrator.

"Old men forget", wrote "a man of advancing years" who resigned over Munich. "The appeasement policy culminated in September 1938"?[2] In March 1939, market forces plead aggressive defence strategies, except when the risk is of "unnecessary war". "The appeasement policy culminated in" "a golden" reference to "Europe, Chamberlain, Daladier, Hitler and Stalin", prior to the occupation of Prague:

> "I consulted Chamberlain on the line that I had better take. His comment was that I should discourage the view that war was inevitable, and insist upon the great possibilities of peace."

"You [Chamberlain] did your best to avert it – far more than any other man would have dared to do."[3]

---

[1] "Corner farm" replies to Robert Ewing
[2] Ian Kenneally (2017)
[3] Geoffrey Dawson (1940)

"'If at first you don't succeed, try, try, try again.' That is
what I am doing." Only the "Foreign Office, certain that it would
be blamed for events over which it had no control, parodied it
cynically as: 'If at first you can't concede, fly, fly, fly again'."

"At Munich we lost a unique opportunity of easily and
swiftly winning a war that was in any case inevitable." "But how
could I have done otherwise? Every one of my single conditions
were met."

Thus Chamberlain has not been blamed for events which
he could not control, but for events which he did control; as
if powerlessness must be considered the consequence of not
appeasing the professional - however "biased". "You and I will
be dead in three months time." That was appeasement. And
such is wrong bias, that notion: "an understanding of that most
astounding and troublesome of all phenomena, human society".[1]
Confusion is the most astounding and troublesome of all
phenomena; and such was the common relation against which
Chamberlain remarked: "All this will be over in three months."
That, as Churchill thought, was not appeasement, however
paradoxical to subsequently declaring "peace for our time".

"Old men forget", but History driven to counter the bias
of blame would conclude that Chamberlain's policy was not
a jack-high-bury wood exploited by the blame-game, rather it
was what the Old remember of their matches: "History smiles at
all attempts to force its flow into theoretical patterns or logical
grooves; it plays havoc with our generalizations, breaks all our
rules; history is baroque."[2]

---

[1]   Kingsley Davis (1949)
[2]   Will and Ariel Durant (1968)

JR /Ewing

"...steeled to barbarity by the cries of the orphans
and the tears of the widows it has made."
Robert Emmet to Green street courthouse

Tom Wintringham – Aberfan remembered certainly but the most important lesson not to trust the kingdom and the royals has not been learned.

If anyone protests dangerous practices of management then very often the kingdom will allow its police officers to arrest that protester so as to allow management peace and quiet to go on risking lives.

The royals cannot be trusted because they prevent any better elected head of state a president of a republic insisting that the state does not arrest protesters for doing their duty to try and save lives.

So the Queen cost the lives lost at Aberfan and the appropriate thing to do was to hold the kingdom itself to account, ending the kingdom, establishing a republic and never again inviting any royal to anything except to leave the country, never to come back, never again to endanger the lives of innocents.[1]

Robert Ewing to Tom Wintringham – Child royals were executed by Russian republicans, and many nuclear weapons on

---

[1]   October 23rd 2016 to thesun.co.uk

from there is the proposal to deactivate the royals connected to the negligence that caused Aberfan. I guess wishful thinking was part of the negligence, and you would perpetuate it, rather than give children a voice against you monstrous adults, squabbling between yourselves even despite the nuclear weapon age, as if you monstrous adults have not cost enough child lives by executing one idea after another.[1]

Robert Ewing – The name of one of the one hundred and sixteen children lost was "Michael Collins". "In a hundred years or more people may be saying that republics were the worst form of tyranny." And it is the worst form of tyranny that those who have most to lose relative to war, while more threatened relative to wars, are not more generally considered as "the lives of innocents".[2]

Robert Ewing – "Many unthinking people in this country, because they do not trouble to picture to themselves how a theory would appear in practice, assume, for instance, that if the coalmines or the railways were 'nationalized', made the property of 'the State', they would become the property of 'the people', that Jack Robinson, travelling third-class to town in the nine-fifteen,[3] would be able to say to himself, 'Well, at all events this train belongs to me'."

That protester, Douglas Reed, June 1942.[4]

---

[1]   December 15th 2016 to thesun.co.uk

[2]   July 3rd 2017 to thesun.co.uk

[3]   The hour and minute of the Aberfan accident

[4]   August 2nd 2017 to thesun.co.uk

The Decisive Battle:
WATERLOO

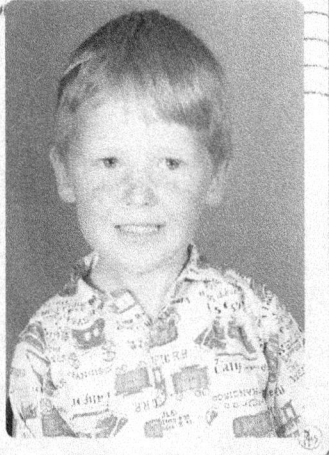

© Edit. Thill, S.A., Bruxelles Tel. 344.92.40

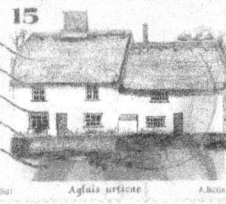

BELGIE·BELGIQUE   15

Aglais urticae   A.Buzin

William Ewing
Abbey Ville House
Kilnadema
Loughrea
Co. Galway

Rep. of Ireland.

The Decisive Battle:
WATERLOO

"Hard pounding this,
gentlemen; we shall

see who can pound

the hardest."
          Wellington
          June 18th 1815

© Edit. Thill, S.A., Bruxelles Tel. 344.92.40

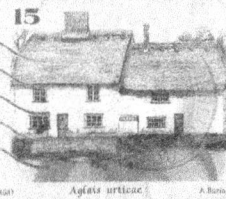

BELGIE·BELGIQUE   15

Aglais urticae   A.Buzin

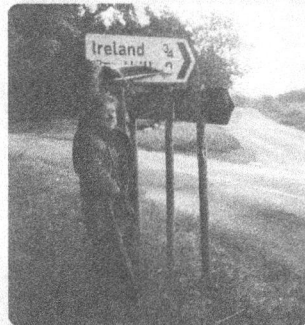

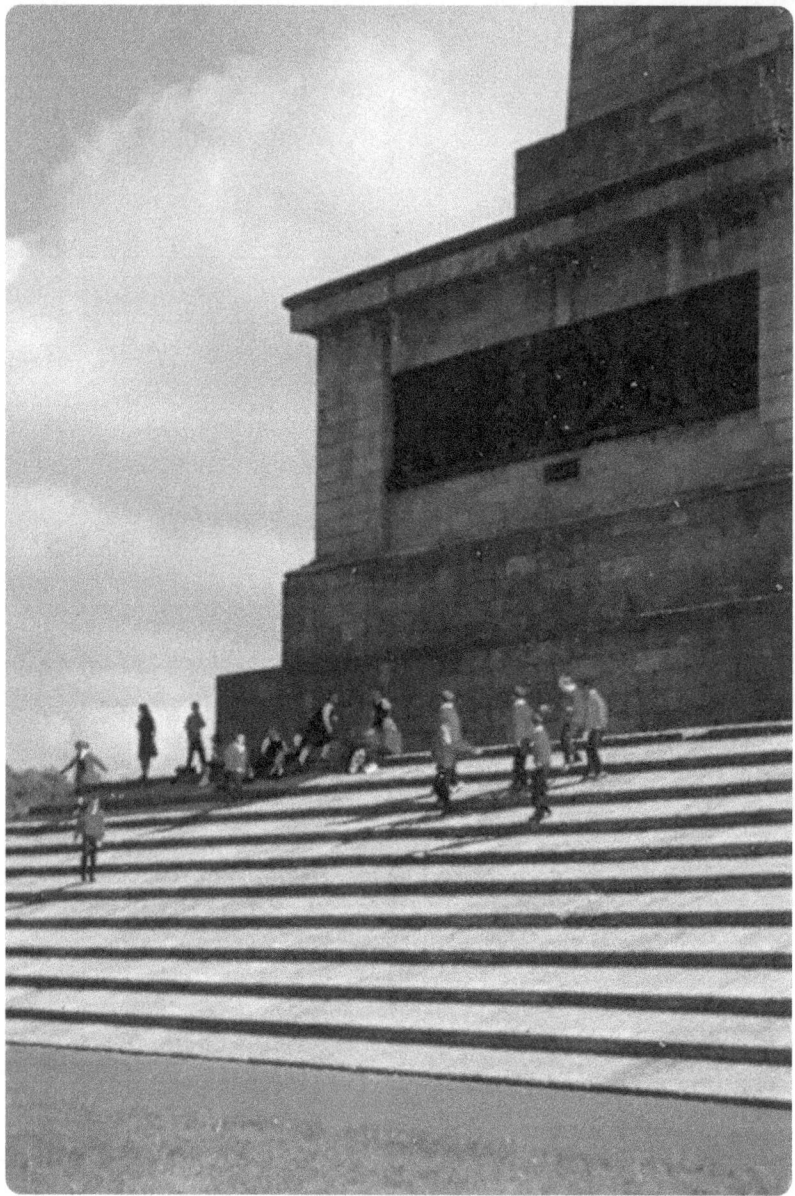

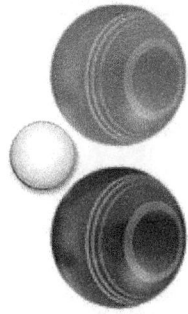

The Crookedness of
Irish Politics

History explains our political parochialism

Gunning for ideas - crooked enough article too, though incisive in places, and sometimes even brilliant

doofus 2016 – I agree the want of direct talking, indeed seriousness, common in many parts of Europe, results in stasis and ill-equips us for the long-term. He doesn't offer solutions, buyt I spose he doesn't have to. Who is he?

ValerieMcDonald – crooked as in warped more than corrupt

MatCon – I've always thought that Ireland has too many politicians. We have 158 TD's compared to the UK's 664! So Ireland has 1/15 of the population but ¼ of the no of TD's.

An old friend of mine who always voted Fianna Fail at one time voted Fine Gael. The Fine Gael candidate got in by 1 vote! My friend proudly boasted that his vote elected the Fine Gael candidate. Where virtually every constituency depends on minimal votes (transfers) to get the last few candidates elected, local issues take precedence over national. A TD who offends an individual/family/community risks not getting re-elected. Tough decisions don't get made, short-termism becomes prevalent.

This situation will never change because who is going to vote themselves out of a job?

Robert Ewing – Why not have your readers provided with the protection to the virus "parasite" – rather more serious than the virus "native" or "coloniser". After all, the State is, and the people are, supposed to be a many splendid thing. Protection means making the most sense in the most appropriate direction, and acknowledging of course the call to bring down the virus.

Equality and Human Rights Commission

Ambition and courage are not to the fore in the IHREC [the Irish Human Rights and Equality Commission]

colour orange – The country only understands civil and political rights. No significant players understand economic and social rights. And it's all about freedom certainly never about equality

two ronnies – Yeah, the language used indicates the government just wasn't into it

natkingcola – So what about the theory we live in the capital of inequality. Human rights that's a different thing and we're much better

Robert Ewing - Human rights through the law is something of a contradiction in terms. Does anybody need to be a rocket scientist to work this out? The legal profession cannot find fault with itself – what a catch!

1916 /ongoing danger of conservative revolution

[An opinion that centenary bouquets lacked the aroma of new ideas]

Revolving Staircase – Couldn't agree more – the whole thing has been more heat than light. When we see little Englandism over there we despise it – Brexit, UKIP, Boris effin Johnson we hate it. It has been central to our own celebrations. So what is the Big idea???

Robert Ewing – Colonialism? That was the tune when the common-man in Ireland was poor - the tune of the Limerick Soviet. Will the 1916/17 establishments not revise their account and consider 1914-18 as a result of rivalry, not imperialism?

Joe Rooney to Revolving Staircase – What is Little Englandism? You mean the suggestion that Britain should have control of its own affairs? Do some thinking rather than sticking empty labels.

Robert Ewing to Joe Rooney – Or what is Little Irelandism – Ireland should have control of its own affairs presumably. August destiny as of Ireland as a great power yet parochial would produce that term, but is there any difference between the potential or actual isms, except the more powerfully supported parochial vision is likely to have the more serious consequences?

Robert Ewing to Revolving Staircase – The late popular historian and socialist A.J.P. Taylor wanted to end authorities as we know them. The exit-Europe campaign seems more direct perpetuation of the negation and control of the individual by institutions.

Now not Then

What a 2016 Proclamation would look like

Jacobin – This is the only relevance of 1916 – what it can say, however primitively, about today. Everything else is completely irrelevant.

Robert Ewing – Is this "original wording" as originality; reference to subsequent declaration;[1] "tribute" concerning form, or even neither entirely one nor another? Certainly no "tribute" can go to form, because "the original wording" concerning the part you quote[2] continues: "oblivious of the differences carefully fostered by" etc. The wording[3] is that the authorities purposefully obstruct the necessary ideals of the population; thus communicating declaration of war as war is commonly declared – with a not entirely fair, even partly absurd, summary of origin. Had the wording been that the highest authorities could not be trusted to oversee fair distribution of power and wealth in Ireland, the document would have had mature teeth.

---

[1]   Reference to the constitution of 1937
[2]   "The Republic ...cherishing all the children of the nation equally..."
[3]   Reference to the proclamation of 1916

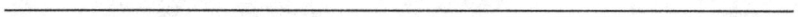

I'm unselfish;
you're selfish

People believe themselves to hold unselfish values but, due to media and politics, inaccurately that others hold selfish ones

Robert Ewing - Confusion is hardly surprising. Identify the common interest: to be informed that an allegation is (or was) made against a State component; or informed that a claim is (or was) made that there is (or was) evidence of component failure? The State system was created to hold individuals to account without specific procedure for processing claim allegations against system components, none of whom provide equalizing specific. That has to change because Bagehot[1] was right: "Protection is the natural inborn creed of every official body; free trade is an extrinsic idea, alien to its notions, and hardly to be assimilated with life". Since the system cultures find it difficult to find individual good deed, we need to create equalizing specifics to key-in 'free trade', whether as incorporated in legal process or as a published report (rather than invite the routine contradictions: "there simply is no legal 'right answer'. But ...an enforceable bill", and/or "take

---

[1]   Walter Bagehot (1872)

more care in defining" constitutional specifics).[1] Thus define
State accountability as the right to know, requiring equalizing
specifics – procedure providing the right to know and equality,
over the 'protection' culture that effectively blocks and distracts
media reporting, thereby controlling the image of business
and component culture at the expense of society generally; the
culture will say: "blames", or: "not supported by any evidence";
and there is evidence that it does.[2]

---

[1] "Politics is key" /"Equality is key"
[2] The Supreme Court 2013 /2001

Is equality a right?

Politics is key, as constitutional rights have served the elite /Equality is key, and best enshrined as a constitutional right

maoliosa – Generates questions about nature of rights but also the key question of whether equality can be a right – and if so what breed of equality can be a right

Robert Ewing - First teacher, then employer, reward performance. Those who teach or employ are rewarded. Trade is the consideration. Rights, while they receive memorable rhetoric, do not represent trade, and therefore tend to receive less reward. Yet equality with the trade culture will not be achieved by definitions, rather only by ensuring that the administrative system works. In other words, accountability is key.

O'Murchú – one of the key discussions. For me equality not a right. Simply, too many people don't want to be constrained by their alleged equality with others.

Robert Ewing to O'Murchú – The question of "alleged equality with others" may be "one of the key discussions" – equality must be about social order, but competitiveness, rather than idealism, tends to be 'the name of the game', and without concern to be fair to others the question of equality is denied positive relation. My conclusion is that there are "too many people" inclined to convince themselves that they qualify for something either equal to or above others, as if appreciating/respecting others is to constrain, rather than perform, order. Fairness should be one of the key discussions, and should be given greater priority in schools, rather than competitiveness encouraged as it is.

Irish poets
learn your trade

On being thought an idler by the noisy set

Dozey – there really isn't any evidence the poetry set have anything to contribute to contemporary Ireland you know, Frank

Robert Ewing to Dozey – Poetry there really is. Killeenadeema-Aille History & Heritage has chairman's introduction referring to the local "personalities of national importance"; and he also provides a specific introduction to my poetical narrative referring most notably to the GAA: "MacLiag, a poet to Brian Boru". Belmont Bowling Club's President of 1884[1] was "Robert Ewing". No tyranny will ever destroy us.

Robert Ewing – "Poetry made prose at Drumcliff" (Village, May 20th 2011): "You could put your foot on the grave and leave the other one rooted in the car-park." You could put your finger on something too. August 31st 2017 to Village: "particularly as concerns emergency exit drill" – "the first rule of Britannia", which prior to the Vegas concert shootings I quoted and indisputably then footnoted at "the pope": "Last sailed at dusk, February 28th 1942" (sunk the following day). Stephen Roskill

---

[1]   The founding year of the Gaelic athletic association

(1960): "Pope, U.S. destroyer, loss of" ("American", indeed); Correlli Barnett (1991): "Pope, HMS (destroyer)" – "sunk" (no such HMS). The resting place for any poet's finger is on the pulse, as it was prior to the murder of MP Cox too: "The late popular socialist..."[1]

Robert Ewing – "The late popular historian and socialist..." Intuition is defined as "the power of the mind by which it immediately perceives the truth of things without reasoning or analysis" /"immediate knowledge in contrast with mediate". History (the conservative) and sociology (the socialist): "port and starboard step successively, and nothing intermediate except ceding identity to the first rule of Britannia" – immediate knowledge in contrast with the power of the mind. The late popular sociology...

Indeed, "Irish poets learn your trade": "the truth of things without reasoning and analysis"; the pulse.

---

[1]   Quotation error: "historian and socialist"

Imagine

Ireland and its intellectuals should embrace symbolism and poetry, even in politics

Robert Ewing – Centuries of "trial"[1] does not presumably claim "colonialism". Try 'religious, political and strategic' considerations for those enigma variations, and create your poetry from there. Shelley drowned in Ireland. Imagine Brian Boru and poet MacLiag walking beside a stream at their level. The king asks about the poets inspiration. The poet is closest to the stream, and falls in up to his crown. However, the king immediately pulls him out, and the poet, dripping from head to foot, answers him: "Ireland has answered your question." Ireland has more answers, but they are nothing without the questions.

Robert Ewing – "Imagine There's a Heaven"?[2] "Imagine there's no Heaven"? October 21st 1805: "It does not signify which" /"take your choice"; neither Murray nor Lennon but Baldwin had the answer, as Aitken related to "The World at War": "Stanley Baldwin didn't give up his gates."

---

[1] Constitution preamble (1937)
[2] John Murray (2017)

Stalin/out

**The world needs more Gorbachevs –
leaders whose weaknesses reveal an
optimistic belief in human nature**

Robert Ewing - "Have all the key-people got stop-watches?"
"Issued them today."[1] Stopping[2] at "eleven minutes" instead of
fifteen meant fear levels had to rise, but imprisonment on what
grounds – the "universal" justification (and favourite allegation of
national courts): money? How might Viktor Suvorov[3] have ticked
that box: 'Have all the University people got stop-watches?' "The
world needs" benevolent warning ("rivalry" – "likely to have the
more serious consequences" – "The late popular …socialist"), not:
"I was taken …by what I assumed to be storm-troopers straight up
to Hitler's chalet …and was proceeding in leisurely fashion to get
myself out of the car" ("I happened at the time to be Master of the
Middleton Hounds, and in that capacity received an invitation").
Halifax not only had "an historical amnesia" concerning the Allied
crisis of May 1940, but held to his "on the way back to Calais"
diary (he would not relate that he began to pass his hat to Hitler):
"I assumed this was a footman who had come down to help me out

---

[1]   Writers Jay and Lynn
[2]   The director of a paper factory ceased applauding at a soviet conference
[3]   Author of Icebreaker (European war a cornerstone of Stalin's policies)

of the car and up the steps" – "Hitler invited …this opportunity. I hoped it might be the means of creating better understanding …if we could once come to a fairly complete appreciation of each other's position" /"He did not challenge this and said that formal agreement between the four Powers might not be very difficult to achieve." Politically, the policy-chief was to 'carry the can': "Chamberlain himself was careful to avoid saying or doing anything likely to cause me embarrassment" – "I only recall one occasion …which I thought …was capable of making trouble"; Mr Chamberlain had no University, and therefore "made no effort to conceal his feeling" politically (his only remaining insecurity being a semi-retired dragon who disliked his forehead).[1] Halifax had been chancellor of Oxford University since 1933, and pointed out that Chamberlain, 'the director of a paper factory', "once got so far as to agree" with him.

Agree with who? Hitler may have been destroyed by his invasion delay of 1941; otherwise by Munich (as he said), and/or the defeat of France in a few weeks – so perturbing Halifax and Attlee of course that they exchanged telephone-numbers (Oxford 406-453).[2] Thus recognise Attila's tick: "The speech, however, was never made …and thus phrases not less than policy were his undoing." In other words, pass him your hat[3] – 1934-1940 ultimately brought down "the two monsters".

It also happened that 'the Master of the Medmenham Hounds'[4] had this note concerning "the War Office" during Halifax's meet there: "those now in power at the War Office liked

---

[1]   David Lloyd George
[2]   Born/died
[3]   Subsequently the subject writer related that he educated in Oxford
[4]   Basil Liddell Hart

to pretend that everything was in a perfect state. They formed a mutual admiration and truth-concealing society" – "the tendency to varnish" /"in general the public were not being properly awakened to the situation"; Lenin could have no doubt guessed their justification: "everything is connected to everything else".

Thus fear levels/stop-watches "out"; Dorothy[1] (and "the Transition Period" for children, between parents and State – the "once got so far as" fifteen minutes), undone. The eleventh day of the eleventh month of 1918,[2] and eleven minutes was too timely indeed without a stop-watch.

Robert Ewing – America was attacked in 1941 without declaration of war. Apologise "for the terrible things they did"[3] as a result, since the motivation involved impressing Stalin (allied to USA, not Japan)? A conclusion of yours subsequent to my comment states: "Oxford thinking alienates too many. If England is to flower Oxford must popularise." I state elsewhere:[4] "Statehood began" /"Education, arts and culture began to flower", and "…if population fear levels in relation to their authorities are instructive as most generally communicating commonsense, not ignorance." Your conclusion relates attitudes as existed hundreds of years ago; not long after which many people had reservations such as you have: "The case …suggests that intellectual progress does not dovetail with moral development."

Populations "alienated from the elite, from the rarefied, educated establishment with all their logic and polish"? The

---

[1]   Replied: "Issued them today."

[2]   The eleventh hour too…

[3]   John Devlin (2003)

[4]   To 'Culture is ethics not just aesthetics'

tatty boots of some ignorant person 'walking over' you is surely
not significant. Universities are supposed to create elites, and
it is generally accepted that power is for elites. A.J.P. Taylor
alleged the authorities to be thieves; and it is generally accepted
that power often corrupts. The polished shoes of some educated
person 'walking over' you is significant as communicating
"cheek & nerve" – power generated 'liberty'. If only our
authorities would apply the opportunism that typifies police-
work – once decency is offended, or the evidence is sufficient,
the suspect is arrested – Taylor's suspect, an elite, arrested.
Instead, the public are almost invariably 'on the receiving end',
and there are numerous examples of elites who only exploited
"exquisite opportunity" to be honest about 'our' circumstances
when they themselves were 'on the receiving end' of the "cheek
& nerve". Their governmental theoretic was no-longer "money"
then, but that someone was 'walking over' them with "polish".
I related the question of honesty to you by way of reference to a
controversy involving a former chancellor of Oxford University.
1941, honestly: who attempted to 'walk over' who? Hiroshima:
"clear moral lines"[1] /"enough is enough"? And Nagasaki?
Perhaps president O'Truman joined judge Norbury for a drink
'too many', rather than invariably adhered to "clear moral
lines": "Being a republic is not, in itself, a guarantee of social
justice or even of basic decency"[2] /"That wretched anarchy
inconsistent with all social happiness and genuine liberty which
they call 'a republic'"[3] – consider them Hiroshima and Nagasaki
respectively, but without 'Bloody Sunday' 194One.

---

[1]   Quoting from 'Stalin/out'
[2]   Fintan O'Toole: "enough is enough" (2010)
[3]   Trial of Robert Emmet (1803)

Culture is ethics
not just aesthetics

Arts and culture supplement the deficits of politics and economics, should be relevant, participatory not consumerist, and generate empathy

Darina Daly – Who says? Culture's value is intrinsic

totus tuus – The big divide is between those who think the arts are about enfranchising the disenfranchised and those who want only artistic excellence.

Robert Ewing – Statehood began as security for "improving the quality of life" (the alternative security was to live "at arm's length"). Education, arts and culture began to flower, and with a more peaceful world have inevitably begun to challenge the State. You say:[1] "then arts and culture must consciously pick up this challenge." Education must too: "The State system was created to hold individuals to account";[2] "a new lens" for art and culture would be to exploit that strength, rather than weaken it by 'playing into the hands' of its failings: "Protection is the

---

[1] Concerning safeguarding or achieving "an ethical" State
[2] Quoting Robert Ewing to 'I'm unselfish; you're selfish'

natural inborn creed of every official body; free trade is an extrinsic idea, alien to its notions, and hardly to be assimilated with life" /"It is an inevitable defect, that bureaucrats will care more for routine than for results" /"Men so trained must come to think the routine of business not a means, but an end – to imagine the elaborate machinery of which they form a part, and from which they derive their dignity, to be a grand and achieved result, not a working and changeable instrument."[1] The failings will send the system increasingly 'off the rails' as it encounters and resists "the shift to participation". Many, and very generally in Ireland, have the State "at arm's length" - the 'old lens' of individually attempting to avoid its failings. Whatever about the State's participation in that culture, such weakness should be "attacked" because it fuels the State's belief in its 'old lens' – that of "grand and achieved result". Accountability is thus "bridge to a civil culture" – the "key" to "a civil society". Ethics are of course more honest than aesthetics, and the institutions have "trapped" more aesthetics than ethics if population fear levels in relation to their authorities are instructive as most generally communicating commonsense, not ignorance. History "is ethics not just aesthetics", and "should be relevant": evolution developed that which we have at arm's length (the hand) with a security mechanism: the tail. Combine the strengths and new-lens the high-jump: bananas will out-live nation States - even if the participatory "proposition represents as much a challenge for the arts and culture sector as for the State."

---

[1]   Walter Bagehot (1872)

New Constituti-on/off

We need to change specific provisions, and restraint of judicial interpretation

Robert Ewing - "Above all we need a constitution ...which mandates judges to grapple with questions of social and economic justice"? Above all the constitution defers to Roman Catholic "obligations",[1] and mandates judges to grapple with questions of social and economic justice. Above all eliminate the controversial hype,[2] and simplify the text. I correct "declaration of aims" as I corrected the Chief Justice and Supreme Court: "social order is the law" (performance care-level identifies order) - "the document" (transitionally referring to Ireland and its foreign relations) has but one aim - "true social order". The text confuses.

Judge explanations for lawyer performance inadequacies are evasive (if only the common barrister-on-the-bench reaction) - a 'public relations' to legal academics in order that they

---

[1] John Coakley: "there was a widespread acceptance among Irish catholics of a version of Irish history that associated British rule with evil, and that largely ignored such material benefits as it had brought."

[2] British rule having insufficient resources to buy-off the independence movement, treaty was agreed, but subsequently it was largely ignored, and the dominant religious ethos of the independence movement would claim, effectively, that the insufficient resource was of "all authority".

continue to believe in the present system ("Messrs Byrne and McCutcheon in this book, make a valiant effort"): "ignorance of the law is compounded by a suspicion and fear that springs from our history" ("Shakespeare ...as was his practice ...had several words for it" - "one of the rabblement said..."). "Confidence mustn't be eroded."[1]

Presidency as you propose seems likely to result in idealism, and in any case generally to friction and division. Irish "unity" may be inevitable, but "order" and "concord established with other nations" are generally elusive, and "the dignity and freedom of the individual" another world, particularly because legal professional indecencies continue despite that ideal.

A new text is inevitable, but to what degree should the legal academic claims of inadequacies persuade, when they principally target the document, not performance? Of course the text should make as much sense as possible, but while legal professionals sometimes intend and achieve as much, legal sense from client and/or litigant is not generally accepted - components generally generate a 'convenience-to-themselves' culture (even the Land Commission accepted solicitor explanations, rather than perform independently and find the fraud against them. "You don't make enquiries of that sort in the City; they seemed like decent chaps; and decent chaps don't check-up on decent chaps to see if they're behaving like decent chaps.").[2] "We need" procedural safeguards; eliminate the 'decent chaps' equation that there is no need for equalizing specific; target the dated system: if true social order diminishes Latin wealth, and has at least been attained in the highest office because Caesar occupies it,

---

[1] Writers Jay and Lynn

[2] Writers Jay and Lynn

he does not survive the senate; officers on the Western Front had to implement some rather idealistic orders, during which they relied on their hand-gun for protection against their own men; and garbage (whether enacted by "the people" or not) provides rats with both cover and nourishment. Understand that solicitors engage in legitimate deceit (such as bluffing client readiness to institute proceedings). Illegitimate deceit is as common ("So the ideal is a firm which is honest and clever?" "Yes; let me know if you ever come across one, won't you?"),[1] and to degrees that the profession will not relate. A reporter commented (and suppose why): "It's all a con, isn't it?" Because most clients and/or litigants cannot cope with the wrongful use of legal professional skills. And not only do solicitors have too much say, the minister has the same deferential relationship to deceitful judgments as the judges have. Human Rights meant less acknowledgment of needs, and more invention of wants. The Clare Champion published my letter about "reform of the legal routine"; it was the February of Jimmy Smyth's passing.[2] "Beware the ides of March"? Heed the Champion, rather than the trends and, "dare I say", the senate; "rights driven" is 'Jimmy Smyth'; 'driven off' is what 'he' gets for valiant effort – the question is not so much that the law needs revision, rather legal thought should cease being the monopoly that it is, even if it means another world to some.

Robert Ewing – You subsequently refer to judge introduction in legal textbooks as "probably written over a bottle of wine".

---

[1]   Writers Jay and Lynn

[2]   I had not heard of his passing, yet the Champion preceded my letter with a poem to him and ended the letters page thus – "Gulliver" had travelled to graduate with a degree in philosophy and a masters on 'The Poetry, Songs and Recitations of the GAA in Munster'

I said: "Understand that solicitors engage in legitimate deceit", and system "as you propose seems likely to result in idealism". I think your statement not only has the level of non-seriousness necessary for such deceit, but seems likely to result in idealism. It seems to me that the Judges with the better reputations are asked to write such introductions, and receive honour thus from the legal academics. The introduction I quoted alleged Irish lawyers to "take refuge in an unthinking and uncritical citation of precedent". However, I explain your lack of seriousness to derive from lawyer dependency on the authority of the court. If the entirety of the public was like me, the court would have no authority over any member of the public, and work for you, as a lawyer, would probably be scarce. I say "probably" legitimately, but yours, as might be expected of the so-called 'public authorities', is a label.[1] Irish law says that I have authority over the Irish 'public authorities', rather than they have authority over me, because my performance care-level is the higher. It is exceptionally high because of my greater understanding of human society, which I achieved by way of attending agricultural college abroad, rather than here. An Irish hotelier with a barrister daughter claimed the legal profession to be "a closed-shop". Lawyer deceit enabled court orders against me, effectively without hearing, as the question was whether or not the 'public authority' has authority over me, and the lawyers did not care to test their 'probably' equation. Such is the "one case", such as you relate with reference to "threat" and "a seedy alehouse" – the profession runs our lives, and the State supports the conclusion that the Irish people do not call for choice such as I obtained – there is the law on the one hand, and the Irish State

---

[1]   Previously: "probably Ireland's leading Constitutional expert"

on the other. Democracy allows the principle that the people should know their options, no-matter if only one person chose differently than the rest; but the State would rather be the end than any means to any end, and that means lie after lie after lie from the courts, which the minister and the public and the media are supposed to accept because higher performance care-level supposedly prevails from the 'public authorities'. The public has a right to know: the courts claim that the legal profession and I have absolutely nothing in common, as I related to my father: "It is the legal profession or Robert Ewing. It cannot be both it appears." There was subsequently no appearance in court on my behalf – client instructions meant nothing, as 'the powers that be' go about denying the Irish people the democracy that they need.

Culture bids can
be about change,
not money

The three Irish contestants for EU [the European Union] Capital of Culture 2020 are top-down and inadequately focus on culture as an agent for transforming people

Robert Ewing – Some things are meant to be – consistency. You can't formulate to state 'can't' in a formal paper. Informally, you could write "can't", and again (since some things are meant to be) "can't" – as you have written. And you subsequently write: "cannot" – correct for a formal paper, and contrary indeed to the language basic that some words re-occur because some things are meant to be. A tribute to Arthur Neville Chamberlain: "consistency and logic"; or simply state his initials[1] and thus summarise your bid for "change" and "solidarity" as "of development" to rainbow-warrior resist the convenience culture of "top-down" and its ecology of excluding the individual case.

---

[1] Reference to the African national congress

INTERLUDE

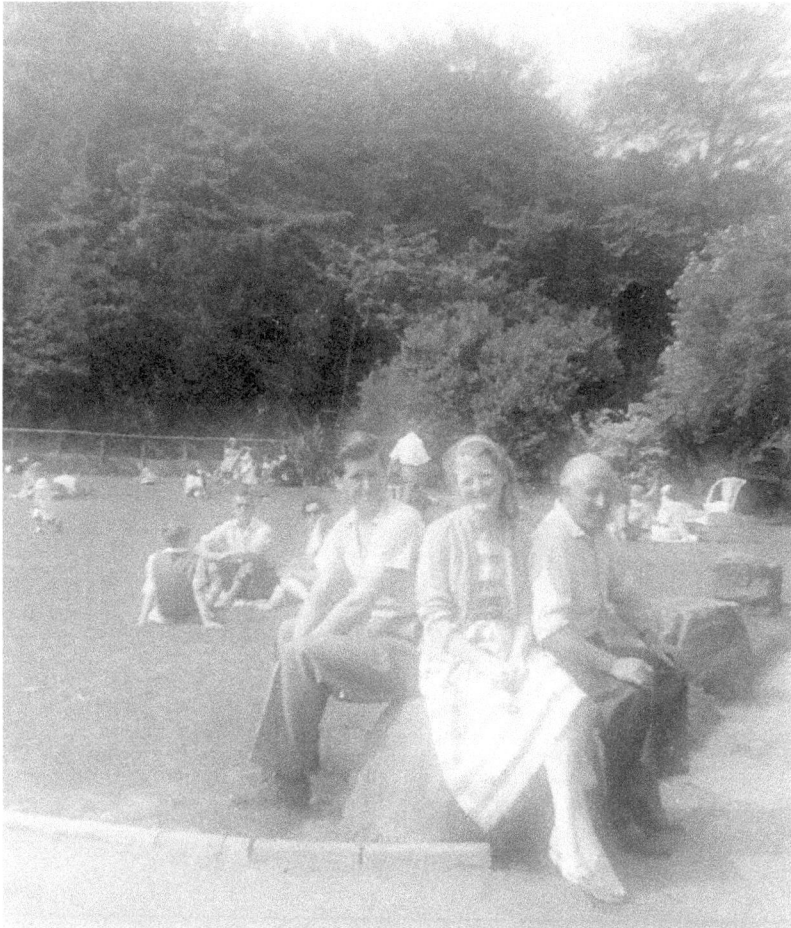

LIFE IS A JOURNEY . . . .

MAKE A NOTE OF IT . . .

Bill,

I called today
to see how you are.
Hope all is well with you.

I am now living in
a village called Marchington
near Uttoxeter in Staffordshire
& working @ JCB. excavators.
Don't often come down these
parts so I had to call
by. Best Wishes.

Ian Jones.

(used to work in the Tech
office @ Perkins many moons ago!)

March bad hare day

Gunning for ideas – What is Village's agenda – does the left it recommends voting for include Labour and Sinn Fein. Not clear

Mercury on a fork – a quotation

John Gunning owned seventeen houses and a soap factory in Bowling Green.

Joyce, not chance – a quotation

Nora left Galway in 1904 and while walking along Nassau Street in Dublin she met James Joyce. This was the beginning of a lifelong relationship, including marriage. Joyce visited Bowling Green on a number of occasions in the company of Nora.[1]

Bonaventure – a quotation

[James Pretsell, 1908:] A bowling-green is the place *par excellence* where the motto of the French Republic – Liberty, Equality, and Fraternity – can be most readily realised.

South fork – a quotation

The real answer lies deep within yourself.[2]

---

[1] William Henry (2016)
[2] John Snell - bowl in hand

Whine and shine – a quotation

Mr. [A.L.] Rowse has gathered together various essays which illustrate, concretely and vividly, the English Spirit.

To Miss Bowen, who speaks of Charles I's "kingly looks", it would evidently come as a surprise to know that he was under-sized, had a stammer and a red nose.

Not a dulles moment - with quotations

To Miss Wilkinson, who concluded: "The other old man would have known", it would evidently come as a surprise to know that the other old man, George V, felt "rotten"; there was a triple threat developing: Germany, Italy and Japan, the French divided, the Americans isolationist, the Russians communist, and his media baited for elections - "they fished in troubled waters, but they were also continually trying to make the waters troubled so that they could fish".[1]

Crack in the tea-cup – a quotation

The economic war ended in 1938 with the *London Agreement*, which proved a triumph for de Valera as a negotiator.

At the time of this Agreement the British Admiralty had made no protest at the ceding of the ports, although even then the clouds of war were gathering.[2]

---

[1]   Leonard Woolf (1967)

[2]   Hally, Éire education (1969)

Don't bat an eye – a quotation

[G. P. Gooch, M.A.] It is the achievement of Bloch and Norman
Angell to have shown that even a successful conflict between
modern States can bring no material gain. We can now look
forward with something like confidence to the time when
[Published *1911*] war between civilised nations will be considered
as antiquated as the duel, [Revised/reprinted February *1913*] and
when [Third impression March *1916*] the peacemakers shall be
called the children of God.

Firing quad – with quotations

In March 1916, the discussion as to whether the Kaiser might be
hanged after the war had nevertheless to end if the peacemakers
were to be called "the children of God"; but April 1916 differed: "In
the name of God and of the dead generations from which she receives
her old tradition of nationhood, Ireland, through us, summons her
children" ("to arms" /"to sacrifice themselves"); and May chose
"the name of God" over "the children of God": "Terry just turned
up"[1] and G. P. Gooch departed thus 'a sacrifice' to Alderman.

Whine-land outshone – a quotation

[Immanent appraisal of the high-policy response to the German
army re-occupying the Rhineland] …and fearing that opposition
at this stage might only make matters worse.[2]

---

[1] David Lawrence - ball in hand
[2] Hally, Éire education (1968)

Well lit – with quotations

The saying was: "smoke or tears". A house once burnt down because butter-paper was placed on the fire, butterflied up the chimney, and descended from that draw to dry thatch.

However, the saying remains: "smoke or tears". "I had my first lesson ...with undesirable official correspondence. The *Locust* had a crack pulling whaler which had always done well in regattas. We[1] ["asked to take her with us to the *Orwell*, which was refused"] ...changed the boats. Shortly afterwards a letter arrived ...asking why the *Locust* had returned a brand-new whaler to the boat slip. This caused ...some perturbation, so I volunteered to ...put the letter on the wardroom fire and we heard no more about it!"

Bull in a china shop – a quotation

In the west of the continent a still more serious catastrophe took place. The prophet Muhammad founded the religion called *Islam* in Arabia at the beginning of the seventh century.[2]

March good hare day

Padraictheplasterer – You must be out of your mind! Do you have no sense of reality. We need STRENGTH or well go the way of syrisa. Theory for the burdz. Cop on

---

[1] "A.B.C." and "the gunner"
[2] Macalister, UCD

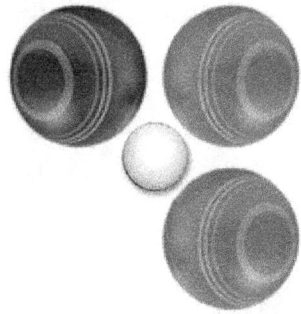

Judicial disappointments

[Book review] A meticulous assessment of the political and discretionary process of judicial appointments [by J. Carroll MacNeil] fails to deliver insider anecdotes

dora at follyfoot – What does morally most wanted mean?[1] The genre is for people who're LEGALLY wanted?

dogears – A little bitchy about this eminent woman, No, Michael?

David langwallner – And where precisely did the assessment of eminence come from

Robert Ewing – A picture such as you lead with should have a government health warning: "They usually all stick together, don't they?"[2] The Phoenix[3] ventured a familiar media approach in April: "he opted to take no further action against the two legal eagles" /"an interesting encounter …with both …expressing deep regret". You venture likewise with your leading picture, despite declaring against media "perpetuation" of circumstances

---

[1] M-m-w, posted 4th July 2016
[2] Writers Jay and Lynn
[3] Current affairs magazine reference to the president of the High Court

such as the following: a lady, allowed on radio about her sensationalist court and newspaper trial, committed suicide. The media may have justification for not astounding the public with what goes on within the legal profession, but there can be no justification for generating public conclusion along the lines quoted: "an interesting encounter". Rising from the ashes: "This book" would have been "an interesting encounter" had it been "the book that needed to be written". And professional 'dirty-work' that breaks the law is rather more newsworthy of course than everyday politics – often involving everyday reliance on public relations such as you suggest an example of.[1]

Village Ed to dogears – Certainly, but overall the review is favourable

Robert Ewing to dora at follyfoot – Yes, the test of performance care-level is with the legal issue – you cannot generate a legal dispute on a moral issue. However, what "morally most wanted" can mean is that the individual particularly concerned with moral issues becomes the "most wanted" as disagreeable to the legal profession; thus did I receive statement of moral issues in case conclusions[2] because whilst the profession clearly prefers to stay away from moral questions, purporting moral issues (such as commonly occurs where "influence" had been contrary to

---

[1]   Subsequently involved with the biased statement concerning the Eire legal system: "There are problems of enforcement" - there are problems with solicitor, barrister and judge availability, and with obtaining that debate, just as there is "everyday reliance on public relations" and "everyday" conclusion consistent with them: "the review is favourable"

[2]   Reference to the lie: "which are clearly of concern to the Plaintiff and are the subject of his complaint..." (2000 /2001)

"the true valuation" of property) can be useful as being contrary to relating true valuation of the injured party – inventing the other party to be "morally most wanted", when truly indeed "LEGALLY wanted". Thus can those with the highest performance care-levels be denied their true valuation, and their influence by way of legal process thereby be obstructed. The profession generally only has one case – every case is treated the same; every word they use is convenient to them.

Robert Ewing to Village Ed – Favourable, while summarised as: "fascinating and meticulous"? Performance care-level summarised as "fascinating and meticulous" is neither "bitchy" nor "favourable", but I do defer to 'two drunks fighting'[1] – I hope neither of you work out who commented.

Robert Ewing to David langwallner – Agus where precisely did the Intermediate Irish History "quick to avail" come from ("The Norman policy was one of territorial expansion and military conquest, and they were quick to avail of the opportunity of invading Ireland")?[2] A registrar at Galway courthouse remarked: "The injustices that go on here!" I heard a lady say to her barrister at the Four Courts: "I think that judge made a mistake?" She had begun to awaken from hers.

Was the concept: "quick to avail", a mistake? Was it serious? That is the question: 'a locality of small farms; an eye over the wall; the opportunity, and the wall is literally hopped over'? Either that is the serious concept of Strongbow's arrival, or we

---

[1] "All drinks are passed by the landlord."
[2] Hally, Éire education (1969)

could call him 'Stringfellow's', or we might ask you:[1] and where precisely is the assessment of eminence going to? We could ask the Law Society, only they have a reputation for 'losing' files,[2] and have been quick to avail of 'the opportunity' to avoid explaining bench appointments with reputation for 'mistakes'. The Society has only 'to ask' the public, or 'to find' a court registrar who, if only on account of his own mistake, had also to awaken from State 'education' and State news such as: "The court heard". How quaint. Because no matter what the courts hear, they have their routine of only one case: part or all of a herd hopped over a wall,[3] thereby (doubtless) quickly availing of 'the opportunity'. Such is the serious cultural debate: was the State's "quick to avail" serious? To say it was means that the religious missionary statement of the Constitution's preamble[4] cannot seem perpetuation of the complained of conquest. To say it was not means that the "quick" was scholarly of the 'Island of Quaints', or simply an every day 'mistake' by the national lie machine. 'We gratefully enact and, therefore, cannot enact a mistake'. That judge subsequently wrote:

> "I have had the benefit of comprehensive submissions from Counsel representing each of the six Defendants concerned and also a lengthy submission partly in written form and partly delivered orally in Court by [the Plaintiff] the Defendant and I am grateful"

---

[1]   Subsequently: "I have cunningly chosen exile, in Prague."

[2]   William Ewing /Barbara Hyland

[3]   Subsequently: "resort to self-help" - reference to solicitor clients

[4]   The review instituted by the State concluded: "overly Roman Catholic and nationalist in tone" (1994)

It is an every day mistake to confuse plaintiff for defendant, and vice versa; it is rather practical therefore to formulate that 'mistake': "the Defendant" ("They're running things for them; for their power, for their convenience, and their benefit").[1] Four of the six defendants were fraud specialist companies, and one of the remaining two was their license provider, the Law Society. And the three further system defendants to those five (also "concerned" not to be ordered against with the non-system 'revenue-head' of the nine), were "representing the State". Mother Shipton (1488-1561) said: "The poor shall most learning know"; but of course the lie machine will 'mistake' the poor for defendants, and simply 'do the hop'.

---

[1]   Writers Jay and Lynn

Judging the Guards

[Éire] Judges and the Garda let our society down: make the Garda Commissioner accountable to the Ombudsman, and establish a Judicial Commission

tad greenway – Wow. This is a wide ranging piece but I'd agree with most of it – all those enquiries to no end

Lucy Byrne – Still. I'd take Ireland any time over what's going on in the US, Britain, France etc. Our democracy isn't fragile whatever Mr Langwallner believes

JimJam – Deference and unction to the judiciary from the media and the politicos

Robert Ewing – You say: "our non-educational results-focused system"; or: 'our education-based qualification non-educational results-focused system'? The dysfunction is rooted in cleverness: European house servants were slaves; those employing them were not servants; the house servants had therefore to liberate themselves.[1] Then, "the Guards" arrive, "not to investigate but to assume guilt", and an anger never heard before announces

---

[1]   The Remains of the Day (1993)

that the root has indeed arrived. The root then encounters the house preservation society; cannot understand its limitations on freedoms, and appeals for liberation again, only this time the servant has a more powerful claim concerning the house: heritage. Barristers are meant to be clever. Education there is, but cleverness does not announce the arrival of the root; and who does, only the leadership of the country[1] – the servants who are means, against whom are the so-called servants who are mean – "they think singularly and exclusively about getting a result, oblivious to any lives they are damaging"? The preservation society certainly has a case against "the Guards", but the root of the problem is that society is letting itself "down" – 'all have the right to be clever', and it trumps all other rights; 'all have the right to be silent', and "the judiciary" like that right the most.

Robert Ewing to Lucy Byrne – He believes: "Standards have certainly slipped. Results have become key and any unethical ruse is tolerated" (Village, October 2016), and I believe that maintaining standards should be based on procedural measures, not on good fortune but on safeguards – his 'safe' Guards, which he believes "a leader with vision and with purpose" such as Obama (posted March 2nd 2017) would contribute, and which I would propose requires a considerably greater departure from the concept that the people get whatever their chance ruler

---

[1] For example: prior to the murder of MP Joe Cox: "Protection means making the most sense in the most appropriate direction" /"Human rights through the law is something of a contradiction in terms" /"rivalry" – "the more powerfully supported parochial vision is likely to have the more serious consequences" /"The late popular ...socialist" /"The exit-Europe..." And prior to the Vegas hotel shootings: "emergency exit" /"American public" – "American public" /loss of "the" USS "pope."

decides, yet not toward his concept that the people can more directly contribute to the legislative process; if his "new Obama" wants the power of the old one, that president might be inclined to maintain the power of those below him, rather than confront the 'I can do anything I want' culture that constantly threatens standards. A strong democracy is not necessarily helpful, as may be believed from your reference to the most famous democracies; the basic of human community, and therefore of any State, is to hear one-another, and it is there that strength matters, not in 'the tyranny of the many over the few' which several parts of Irish society have complained about,[1] and which has been much regretted, not least by the few who note that Ireland might well be termed a village, and who ask how a complex village has had no administrative creativity to contribute. "We need, like the phoenix from the ashes, a new Obama..."? The 'name of the game' here should be 'Ireland', not 'Eire', and from that phoenix administrative creativity might begin to "flow". "Extremism has become normal"? How fragile is the Irish vision when we are all to be dictated to? As fragile as the Irish media allows it to be. We need to know who is doing what to who. We need more than "a new Obama" to enable "our younger generation ...see how" it can contribute;[2] confidence recruits, such as you expressed: "Ireland any time..." Only the intellectual would not have confidence in the Irish State, and that is what was expressed.

---

[1]   For example (an orphan to the Clare Champion, 15th February 2013): "My favourite song is by Gene Pitney, *A Town Without Pity*. It played every Friday night and for me, it sums Ireland up."

[2]   "I have no doubt that many ...have a need, a felt want, to make a contribution and a difference but cannot see how that can be channelled through conventional political structures."

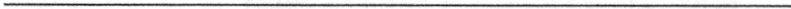

Extremism has become normal

Dump neo-liberalism and build the just society, optimising liberalism and equality envisaged by Rawls, Dworkin and Costello

Robert Ewing - "Only the intellectual would not have confidence in the Irish State,[1] and that is what was expressed." I quote from my comment today concerning this posting and Mr Langwallner's 'Judging the Guards'.

Helen Collins – Yes we have seen some interesting moves in Ireland like the water protest where the neo liberals tried to sell it back to us. Let's hope this is only the start of the fight back

Robert Ewing – "After the presentation a prominent legal academic came up to me" and said: 'While something of a comedian myself, it is something of a privilege to hear a real expert.' "Put people in a box and they will not work properly" ("Alain De Boton argued in 'The Architecture of Happiness'"). "A charmless Irish twist" indeed: De Boton's controversial apologia

---

[1] I notified the president that I had no confidence in the minister for justice or government, and subsequently the deputy prime minister (the Tánaiste) resigned relative to having been minister for justice

for the "black and tans", that some of them had been recruited from prison, and therefore 'did not work properly'. However, as something of a comedian myself, the important point is to join the stigma of prison with British rule. The serious point is that Simon definitely said: "lawyers as a class were often objects of suspicion",[1] but the dregs of society are generally never locked up; they put 'knives in backs' – unlike the "black and tans", for example. "The Architecture of Happiness": "The Neanderthal" male 'lifting his leg' to piss against the wall at the end of his road. It is the pursuit of happiness at someone else's expense, and when that someone else has left the courtroom – his back turned, the lift is secured; and society attaches no stigma to the court for its so-called "Judgement" because it is a 'knife in the back', and who has heard of Alain De Boton anyway, only people who want to work properly? 'Make working properly pay', you said, which to your "considerable surprise, was very well received"; the charmless myth was that Collins was shot in the back.[2] Perhaps we can call a Judgement by a court working properly: 'Towards a West Cork Society'.

---

[1] John Simon to the Canadian bar association, 1921

[2] One theory concluded: "Scotland yard always gets its man."

Adventures in British Imperialism

Books by Urwin, Cadwallader and Cobain illuminate the viciousness of end-of-empire Britain from Ireland to Kenya

John Taurus - My Great-grandfather William Crowell Lonergan was thrown out of Ireland by the British in the late 1800's along with his 16 brothers and sisters. They were loaded onto ships and the captains were told to dump them at the first country in which they arrived. The Demon's that controlled England then still control most of Europe today, including Ireland. These Devil's servants have imposed unlimited immigration from non-White countries into all of Europe, effectively destroying your countries as they have the United States. How many are allowed into Israel, the country that did 9-11 in the United States to set Americans into an Arab killing frenzy and to fight Israel's enemies? It is not popular to say so, but not all people are created equal. That is REALISM not RACISM. Blacks are very low on intelligence and high on violent behavior. It is too late to save Germany. London now has more Muslims than Whites.[1] Ireland is following in those footsteps. Soon, because of rags like the Village brainwashing and steering the sheeple such as

---

[1] February 8th 2017 – subsequent to "Bull in a china shop"

yourselves, you will no longer have a country to call your own. Your daughters will be raped and your sons murdered. If the Jew media published that feces sandwiches are good recycled nutrients, you would stand on the corners gobbling them down. Wake up.

Robert Ewing to John Taurus – On behalf of Village, if I may, I rag you at Oxfam Ireland (.org) contacted today:[1] "I see such television advert for saving lives as decades ago, and question the data presented. I would have more interest in such adverts if there was available to the public a report concerning the record of people lost since the aid began – informing the public of whether there is statistical change over the years; have every death related to us…"

Robert Ewing – At Oxfam Ireland (.org) contacted today: "Following 8/2/2017, Philip Beynon: "I remember driving into the village with him and someone saying if the coal tip behind the village ever came down it would hit the village school." Lack of sense has cost many lives. Where are the statistics and the sense in an apparently unending crisis?"

Robert Ewing – An "unending crisis": 'I can do anything better than you can' – conservative ideology, as expressed in 1969 (Hally M.A., concerning the 'returned' treaty ports, and Collins M.A.): "The economic war ended in 1938 with the London Agreement, which proved a triumph for de Valera as a negotiator." /"What they did not realize was that an older, quite different way of life had been in existence in Ireland for

---

[1]   February 8th 2017 – prior to reading "John Taurus"

many centuries." Judge Niall McCarthy's published foreword said: "most regrettably, attitudes of lawyers in Ireland remain English orientated." Perhaps it is the willingness to make such statements that enables the Irish capital's conservative ideology to survive. 'Lock up your daughters' – "Your daughters will be raped and your sons murdered." My father commented about the capital's conservative element[1] as if to coin a new phrase: 'more English than the English themselves'. That is hardly "an older, quite different way of life", and would likely burn a hole in your pocket. 'Adventures in Irish Conservatism' "from Ireland to Kenya"; make no mistake about it, join Oxfam Ireland instead.

---

[1]   Alleged by Village as "established Dublin families" (March 2017)

Protecting ancient buildings in Ireland: a new initiative

A professional conservation charity focusing on minimal intervention wants to collaborate with Irish groups and seeks prescribed status to comment on planning applications for pre-1720 buildings

Robert Ewing – Considering an individual case: "I can only conclude that our public representatives don't care", "how we neglect our built heritage in Ireland is shameful, and it's very sad." Another conclusion: this 'public representative' cares too much about a symmetrically elegant Irish "Abbeyville House" (a protected structure dated "1820") developed from a pre-1720 "Abbey Ville" – "shameful" and "very sad" to "neglect" nothing of its unique aesthetic impact and 'public representative' family heritage.[1] I care: it would be less shameful and sad to put one's foot through the Mona Lisa. Yet love for the individual, rather than for the artist, is to conclude that our celebration of "curious"[2] should be with the building – what is truly shameful and sad is to refer to the care for the Mona Lisa as more celebratory of art.

---

[1] Most famously involving 3,000 people at both Loughrea and Murphy's field (Craughwell)

[2] "An unusual and curious house" (RPS 3604)

[Taoiseach] Enda Kenny: good for business but not equity and the environment

Robert Ewing – Technically, Kenny's place in history, like Gore's, was decided by the Supreme Court. In October 2013 the Court re-stated the High Court's conclusion that courts may not "direct the government". Firstly, note that courts can only direct relative to themselves; secondly, note that court order provides a choice rather than any direction; and thirdly, note that no such pleading: "direct", existed, the pleading was for an order recommending the government to institute an inquiry concerning Judgment of the Court of October 2001, and those proceedings themselves having connection to previous proceedings. I was not principally concerned to obtain inquiry, but merely for the State machinery to do its job.[1] The case was a procedural inevitability, but the courts effectively attempted to direct the government against considering the issue – the historic event of Kenny's administration was made a non-event; the courts refused to clarify the matter for the government, and simply stated nothing both accurate and significantly relevant –

---

[1] Order "recommendation" to the government was the principal concern, irrespective of whether or not the government would institute an inquiry, as official statement that a number of High Court and Supreme Court decisions are in question, as are the claim results against the Circuit Court defendants in question; both the State and society thus served

the indisputable fault with the Judgment of 2001. Kenny might have been persuaded otherwise to quote Walter Bagehot, and he would have thus obtained "his place in history". He had other things on his mind no doubt, but history may say that he was not inclined to inconvenient truth,[1] and "not quite" Ireland's finest hour is to call to mind Gore's wooden spoon, not the history of Ireland.

---

[1]   He is known to have lied to the Dáil as Taoiseach, as would Tánaiste
     Frances Fitzgerald

Neoliberalism cloaked as modernity

Ireland should brace for market worship dressed up as equality of opportunity and favouring those who [reference to Taoiseach Leo Varadkar] get up early

Robert Ewing - "The dark forces of Neoliberalism have proved very powerful indeed." Consider this: "There was a total absence of tipping policy and this was the basic cause of the disaster." /"There is no legislation dealing with the safety of tips in this or any country, except in part of West Germany and in South Africa." The basic cause of the disaster to Aberfan were "dark forces" beyond "a total absence of tipping policy"; local concern was ignored. While people have their jobs their machinery routinely appears adequate to them, and Village has had that approach: "Hardiman was a master of the truth. One need only read his judgments on our delinquent tribunals and constabulary."[1] Effectively, there is nothing to read: this State journey of ours has no logbook. Dark forces at Aberfan? Neoliberalism? "It isn't hysterical to fear that the end of human civilisation is glaring us in the face". Nothing glares for the

---

[1] Village, April 2017

blind; where is there a State component which reports that a particular document (most importantly: a judgment) simply will not do? Dark force, or is it just pitch-black out there – we are simply running into one-another, not hurling? And the component survivors of this commotion are the clever ones; no judgment serves the people of Ireland which does not forward reform of the legal system; the system survives because it is operated by survivors; and therefore consider them, one and all, our blindness, and the government the dark forces which will not restrain the cleverness of the system profiteers. One need only read: "a system of public plunder";[1] therefore, why not ask the State to give the public something to read, instead of simply running into queer street with nothing more to cover your backsides than a long word and the rosary?

Robert Ewing – "Nothing glares for the blind"; historic Aughrim had to be by-passed, only the hearing for the villagers and village businesses occurred after the proposal was decided; they met with public relations, rather than with anything else. Discovery against solicitors confirmed communications behind several clients backs, as is the practice of towing-the-line that Village has reported[2] and that county council had been involved in, only Aughrim is an innocent example of the daily exploitation of the public's inclination to be entertained rather than informed, as towing-the-line unconsciously is to remain pitch-black rather than evolve into dark force. "Nothing glares for the blind"; ignorance can bring people together, but "a total absence of tipping policy" is no line to tow.

---

[1]   A.J.P. Taylor (1957)

[2]   Village, March 2017: "it is a help to be privy to the corruption."

Cormac O'Neill - As a measure of his originality, let it be remembered that his slogan comes from Sarkozy, La France qui se leve tot.

And as a measure of his understanding of the circumstances of this country, let it be remembered that he wanted to cut public spending by the 80 billion demanded by the troika in ONE year.

Ungenerous Ireland

Economic migrants, refugees, asylum-seekers and asylum-seekers-turned-refugees

Ciaran Caughey – Every last one of them should be kicked off the island. We owe NOTHING to Africa or Asia!

Robert Ewing to Ciaran Caughey – Do you understand what was said? Not one of them "will be able to sue the Irish State" – unless "one of them" has either lawyer training or lawyer experience; professional lawyers, provided every last one of them involved will be paid, are your sewers.[1]

---

[1] October 21st 1805: "It does not signify which" /"take your choice."

Judicial Reform: independence yes; pouting no

archie I, o'chus – Maybe the judiciary should be gotten rid of altogether... after all what truly social and egalitarian purpose does it serve? None so far as I can see. No it exists and always has to look after the interests of the rich, the powerful and the privileged... and if you happen to have been born with a plastic spoon in your mouth, which is most of us, well, hard lines! It won't make any difference, certainly not improve things, by getting in lay people... that amounts to nothing more than tinkering with the works when the machine itself is and has long been at fault, nay redundant.[1] Now if perchance by lay people you mean ordinary people including ex-cons and members of the citizenry who have been on the receiving end of injustice most of their lives then all to the well and good but that won't happen, not in a million years...! No it'll be the same old crowd of busybodies and cap-doffers bowing and scraping before their Royal Lordship Highnesses.

---

[1] Walter Bagehot: "An extrinsic chief is the fit corrector of such errors. He can say to the permanent chief ["idle in real doing"] ..."Will you, Sir, explain to me how this ...conduces to the end in view" ...It is he, and he only, that brings the rubbish of office to the burning glass of sense."

Robert Ewing to archie I. o'chus – I could read your comment as often as one of my own, but I would not read the "hard lines" of the subject itself, as it concerns "the same old crowd of busybodies and cap-doffers bowing and scraping before their Royal Lordship Highnesses", who would be republican to avoid the fraud squad!

The Supreme Court by Ruadhán MacCormac

A racy but meticulous biography of the Supreme Court, its judges and its famous litigants

Robert Ewing – What a wonderful concept: Supreme Court and a biography of it, only when I pleaded the rule of law to the Court there did not seem to be anything between the principal on the bench and the bench. The law belongs to its exponent; and a biography about biographers, while original, is not about the bench.

Robert Ewing - A customer in the Palace Bar said to me that the State-paid individuals involved must think me mad to institute lay-litigant proceedings against the State.

What is mad is that a number of former State defence barristers occupy the bench, few of whom would not have learnt how little the State is concerned with "bringing to life its stories through its judges and litigants". The Supreme Court had produced fourteen pages of lies; and would maintain its story with fourteen more, as a bar-stool thrown professionally always shatters on impact, and therefore a further stool was thrown – the splinter court versus the supremo!

Uncool Britannia

The UK is flouting the obvious lessons and diktats of history and economics

Robert Ewing – Cool Hibernia: human "fodder" and "dangerous fools", "estates" and "Empire". Uncool Britannia: Neville Chamberlain was "more tragic."[1] Is "this Republic" learning anything? Identify the history, and thereby the confusion which you are articulating. Chamberlain and Horace Wilson were not "dangerous fools";[2] so appreciate that Hibernia and Britannia mythologists account for "Donald Trump" and "the Brexiteers". Enda Kenny remarked to the Dáil: "We are all patriots." One might say: "all" Irish; then "who knows why" it is acceptable Irish patriotism to be "riven by" appeasing the culture of opportunism such as produces the "hearts" you call "tragic", rather than accept that Chamberlain moved to stop such "class system" as "is flouting the obvious lessons and diktats of history", by being disinclined to learn anything?[3] Cool Hibernia would conclude that a lot of people will have to revise their historical notions

---

[1]   Village referred to the USA and concluded: "The UK is more tragic."
[2]   Village referred to political developments in the USA and UK
[3]   Questioning Village's neglect to revise Chamberlain's significance

before they can claim association with "mature body politics"; and Chamberlain said that too: "When I was a little boy..."[1]

Robert Ewing – "Britain has struggled with its post-colonialising identity. Particularly" (Intermediate Irish History:) "the British Admiralty had made no protest at the ceding of the ports, although even then the clouds of war were gathering." Six year old children now have their motto: "character is destiny", particularly as concerns emergency exit drill, which is not to 'hop to it', but is port and starboard step successively, and nothing intermediate except ceding to the first rule of Britannia, which is not to cloud the relation between port and starboard, as an adult might fathom the relation between a port and a warship, and the identity of the pope.[2]

Máirtín D'Alton to Robert Ewing – Without an associated airfield the treaty ports were not capable of being defended. The Cumann na nGael government were amenable to leasing land to the British Government to provide air fields for the RAF but DeValera was against it. After DeValera was re-elected the British realized the ports were a liability and relinquished them. That's why the Admiralty didn't object.

Robert Ewing to Máirtín D'Alton – The same historian had written in his European History: "and fearing that opposition at this stage might only make matters worse." He thus spoke some sense about the re-occupation of the Rhineland question which

---

[1] Quotation error: "When I was a boy" /"Little Boy", indeed: "I used to repeat 'If at first you don't succeed...'."
[2] Last sailed at dusk, February 28th 1942

he would not apply to "appeasement" generally.[1] American capital ships had reinforced the blockade against William II; "the Admiralty didn't object"; the British would court American public opinion[2] and would not exclusively depend on De Valera to avoid conflict[3] that might alienate American public opinion – America being the "strategic reserve".[4] Irish military power neither generated partition nor the ceding of ports; my father remarked: "De Valera was a statesman." The myths are "a liability" to everyone.[5] Narrator Andrew Marr remarked: "Chamberlain did nothing."[6] Chamberlain did absolutely everything.[7] He even returned Dev's glasses.

Robert Ewing – "Remember", advised Churchill, "it isn't only the good boys who help to win wars, it is the sneaks and the

---

[1] William Scott (1968): "Munich has become such a damning symbol that the personality and policies of Neville Chamberlain may never be fairly judged."

[2] "I intend to keep on doing everything I can to promote Anglo-American understanding and co-operation."

[3] Chamberlain: "you would have to send troops to protect your rights in the Ports."

[4] Ambassador Ronald Lindsay (1939): "our hidden reserves"

[5] Roy Douglas: "The most powerful arguments against Chamberlain do not really turn on the wisdom or unwisdom of the substantive measures which he took, but rather on the repeated indications that he believed Hitler to be telling the truth." A cousin, concerning Munich: "he didn't believe a word he said…"

[6] Roy Douglas: "The Prime Minister would scarcely have improved prospects for the future [seventh Duke of Wellington] if he had risen in the House of Commons and spoken in terms like these…" /William Strang: "wise to take Herr Hitler at his word when he says that he has no further territorial ambitions in Europe."

[7] "The only hope of doing business with Hitler is to take him at his word."

stinkers as well."[1] Village, October 2017: "May is surely" neither a sneak nor a stinker; as "Uncool Britannia" she patted them on the back,[2] indeed as "Hyacinth" Churchill would, and as such the Village "Bouquet" is more "Bucket" than spade, indeed less terror for the administrative gangsters – competent and correct administration being the spade,[3] and as such no 'Narrator' pat on any Chamberlain back.

[1] To John Dill, October 1940

[2] Conference speech: "Building a country that works for everyone." /Chamberlain: "I am prepared to deal with her on the basis that she means what she says."

[3] "I felt sure it would frighten the totalitarians."

How do the poor die?
We need Orwells, Sinclairs, and LS Lowrys to depict the age of neoliberalism

Do not destroy ordinary humanity: celebrate it

Robert Ewing – "The comments he has made on affidavit are extraordinary", spoke High Court judge (siding with State intimidation via an extraordinary "civil" application); I referred to the bench culture precisely as you relate: "Lowry". Your comments are therefore extraordinary, but you need to quote Neville Chamberlain as relevant case law: "What fools these dictators are!"

Robert Ewing – "Certainly in Ireland there is ...a system descending into anarchy"? Anarchy is a society failing to provide realisable hearing rights, and there is evidence that the Irish State perpetuates the failure (rather than reacts to it), and is not even inclined to react to reports such as yours,[1] as State and business side together (rather than hear the public), as if dreaming of a 2084 when only "our ruling classes" can claim

---

[1]   Previously: "Ireland ...does not as a state conform to the rule of law."

moral or intellectual distinction. In other words, no "ordinary" citizen can generate a public controversy of "a system", even for eighteen and a half minutes, "descending into anarchy", because the anarchists (not simply "wealth and property") "run the country". The public votes for a 2084 in which election slogans mean what they say: "Your President"; yet it may be 2184 before the State accepts the most simple and important test of statehood: realisable hearing rights; until then, it is a fraud that will "go after anyone that poses a threat to" its exploitation of "the ordinary person", who, irrespective of the circumstances, can never find it. Celebrate the day when "humanity" can say: "we found", and the "we found" of "the tactics of surveillance" is dead.

INTERLUDE

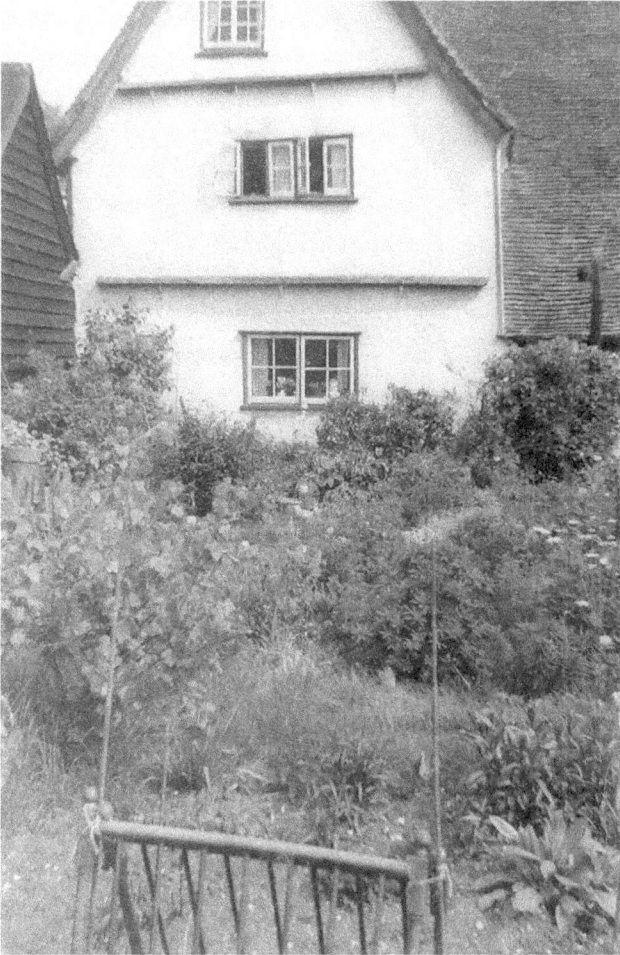

. . . . HOME

Thank You
Robert
Your kind
thoughts
can be put
into action.
     Its possible
since there was
only one person
without sufficient
funds to ask anyone
to pull resources
for this one tired
PERSON.
          from
     Brooke in
the meadow
     200 swagman

Silent worship

dog&bone – Is it the rising that's boring, or the coverage, or what politicians have (not) made of it? Or is it just that the Village is boring?

Just Mary – I think Michael D. was referring to discussions on the Rising rather than general worldwide political discourse being dominated by self-loathing for nationalists, while colonialism in all its guises passes without comment or even recognition

Where there's a will – a quotation

[*Robert Ewing* to Michael ("the thousands of isolated individual cases") D. ("a thousand 'strokes'")[1] Higgins] The 'folklore' is that the local IRA seat (uncle of our opponent) brought legal firm into Loughrea that the IRA elsewhere had objected to. While paranoid speculation about the possibility of spy is somewhat cultural, Clare IRA found a letter in his pocket that caused intention to shoot him. The 'tans' burnt two local IRA houses, and he is the suspect for informing them – 'running with the hare and hunting with the hounds' (he was certainly otherwise a natural choice). He led a failed attempt to get hold of our guns (whether it concerned dispute in 1902[2] or targets were scarce); the police came out that evening for them. Our opponent wanted our lands, and relied on that firm to misadvise my late father[3] – involved there because the Will was.

---

[1] Poverty, inequality and youth unemployment (1983/4)
[2] Concerning claim to divide the dwelling
[3] Prior to Village: "any unethical ruse is tolerated"

No bulletin – a quotation

[Regional newspaper report concerning the District Court and confiscation to the minister] No cert. William Ewing of Killeenadeema West, Loughrea, was given the Probation Act at Loughrea court last week for possessing [volunteering] an [obviously unusable] air pistol and lead pellets without a firearms certificate on April 20th [Easter Monday] 1992 at his home. Inspector Martin Lee said there was no "sinister involvement" in Ewing having the [useless] pistol.[1]

Spanner set and match – a quotation

Irish monasteries were a rich source of plunder.

They were also obnoxious to the Vikings, for they were schools for the propagation of Christianity, a form of religion hateful to the Norse pirates.[2]

Nuts and lightning bolts – a quotation

Early in the sixteenth century a further cause of strife and suffering made its appearance. This was the great religious revolt to which has been given the name of the Reformation.

The Fruit of the Reformation: [Drawn] the Destruction of a Monastery.[3]

---

[1]   Connacht Tribune (1992)
[2]   Macalister, UCD
[3]   O'Mullane, Free State education

Potter's bar – a quotation

Huge respect 4 u guys
ur part of the place
ur dad trusted a thief,
a wolf in sheeps clothing
it shows a very calculated
and manipulative attempt
at stealing another mans
property and whilst he
was sidetracked with a
distressing personal
situation and was[1]
vulnerable And not
thinking clearly

AJP tailored – with quotations

"The Magic Years of Beatrix Potter ...places Sawrey in Cumberland which it never was."[2] Kellogg proposed and signed a multinational treaty renouncing war, in order "to outwit"[3] Briand; thus began "an international kiss" (called the "Kellogg-Briand Pact" or "Pact of Paris"), and the name "William Arthur Pax Ewing", subsequently of 1 Wellesley Terrace, Limerick, and, by treaty "(being sufficiently recommended unto Us for your honesty of life and skill and knowledge in music) to hold and serve the said place" – "vacant by the resignation of Archibald James Potter..."[4]

---

[1]   Kiln-nadeema text messages
[2]   A.J.P. Taylor (1978)
[3]   Robert Ferrell (1959)
[4]   Dean and Ordinary of St Patrick's Cathedral

Village times – a quotation

When you speak of reason presumably you're speaking of the [L] Logus, the [B] Word, the [W] Breath of God.

I[1] think ...Swift (just to name one truly great thinker) got it right when he wrote (in Gulliver's Travels) that lawyers are "a society of men bred up from their youth in the art of proving by words multiplied for the purpose, that white is black and black is white, according as they are paid."

Lee-ward – a quotation

He [the late William Ewing] would have been entitled to a Certificate and we now enclose one. There is a possibility that the National Museum would be interested in the Medal.[2]

Auction this day – with quotation

Churchill volunteered a question at the height of the Battle of Britain: "What reserves have we?" The result was a bi-plane marked "Action this day" and pilot's cap marked "Winston".

Worcester source – quotations

I [J.E.T. Harper, 1927] WANT to make it quite clear... /[Ian Botham - bat in hand] Too many people live in the past.

---

[1]   Archie Lochus to the Washington Times /Village
[2]   Feis Ceoil administrator to Robert Ewing (1999)

Welsh wizard – with quotations

Politics is not "the art of the possible", rather of mumbling –
attempt to have things both ways:

"'Hark! I hear the foe advancing'", mumbled 'Trick, audible as
a dragonfly. /'Mumbling missionaries', mumbled the pope. 'And
how goes it in Ireland?'
    'We've banished the snakes.' /'*We've* banished the snakes?'
    'You've banished the snakes.' /'*I've* banished the snakes?'
    'I've banished the snakes.' /'You've banished *the snakes?*
You've got to get it together, 'Trick.'

In the beginning – a quotation

Report on the first comprehensive [school] year 1970-71

Humanities Department /T. Pope, B.A. [to December 1970]
/Our aims are:

1, To increase knowledge and understanding.
2, To promote interest in the subjects and to foster the spirit of
inquiry.
3, To encourage active participation (e.g. drama, debates, choral
and orchestral work, research, visits).
4, To prepare for examinations, internal and external.

The latest project to be considered by the Community Association
is the possibility of a bowling green. A preliminary meeting will
be held on Monday 19th July.

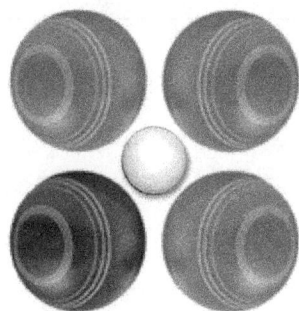

Lowry and Sinclair
[Revised title[1] to:]

Do not destroy ordinary humanity: celebrate it

Robert Ewing – "Neoliberalism..."?[2] Nellie Oleson[3] would "probably faint dead away."

Robert Ewing – You subsequently state that "litigants resort to self-help" because "litigation is often scandalously expensive ... and the wheels of justice move at a grindingly slow pace." You may as well be pleading a case for Oleson's Mercantile against John Ingles, who buys in another town allegedly because of Oleson high prices, delayed provision of goods, and spite concerning Nellie's conflict with his daughters at school. He shops elsewhere because Oleson's is the tyrant of his locality, but they say that farmers bringing livestock to mart are "clogging up" the roads, delaying goods haulage and thereby forcing up prices, and that the dispute is an everyday customer confrontation, except generated by spite; to which the judge concludes with "the favourite allegation of national courts": "money" – Ingle's shops elsewhere to save money.

---

[1] Subsequent to my second comment to "How do the poor die?"
[2] Liberalism suited to free-market capitalism
[3] Unknowing of the controversy or subsequent resignation of Tánaiste Frances Fitzgerald

You say that the alleged money-savers are "clogging up the lists with spurious cases and endless illogical and *de minimis* arguments",[1] but what is "endless" is legal professionals referring to money.[2] Lay-litigants said to me that the lawyers take "control" of the case, rather than further it; the same "spurious" management generated the dispute in which my late father was involved, and continued by way of subsequent companies; "control" of the town; and the "spurious" explanation: "cost". "Stopping at "eleven minutes" instead of fifteen"?

"The list system in the Four Courts is a shambles"; Walnut Grove is a shambles; "ordinary" citizens "resort to self-help" – they pursue money, as that is, effectively, their only voice.[3] "There are problems of enforcement in Ireland." The basic origin of courts of law was to enforce payment to the State, and "enforcement in Ireland" of "the rule of law" for individuals[4] is "scandalously" subservient to the legal professional culture of explaining motivations as I related in Stalin/out: "on what grounds" – "money". Indeed, "the profession only has one case";[5] for example: not everyone has resorted to self-help, or exploit the cultures generated by it; therefore there must be a character reaction somewhere against the "spurious cases"

---

[1]   Robert Ewing, 18th October 1997: "It is quite obvious a very choked court system is well suited to members of the legal profession who wish to manipulate cases and clients away from proper court hearings."

[2]   "Do not destroy ordinary humanity" referred to money as arguably it had to, but the subject writer subsequently otherwise referred to money

[3]   Subsequently, Joyce and Sheridan to the Galway Advertiser: "How they tried to keep you down..." /"to keep people down" (8th February 2018)

[4]   Robert Ewing, 18th October 1997: "For us there is no rule of law in this State. The law is in the hands of a legal club. When one of its members fail to uphold the law in relation to a member of the public (their client) the other members refuse to act against him."

[5]   Quotation error: "The profession generally only has one case..."

generated by the legal profession. Accept that character reaction: six years is "a grindingly slow pace"; forty million is "scandalously expensive"; but the character relating this case says that the "pace" and "cost" was an inevitability[1] of good administration; such is the logic against your conclusion based on the judge's statement: "disputes which the parties themselves are unable to resolve"; one side is able to resolve it but the other side is predatory; one side has the character but the other side is "endless" reference to money; one side is Chamberlain but the other side is dictatorship; one side is Ingles but the other side is Oleson: "I can loan you money if you need it." What is "compounding the problem" is the basic origin of the courts – not "cases" by lay-litigants attempting to avoid Oleson. If you want "wheels of justice", work for character evolution against the common problem that concerns are not for right or wrong but business, and against the routine negation of disputes by the "endless" profession on behalf of Oleson's and the "endless" State.

Robert Ewing – "All God's children have three dimensions, and lives outside of work." Clarkson[2] /May: my second comment concerned the subsequent statement by this subject writer and could not be found subsequently until I re-typed it to the posted new subject;[3] disquis mistakes that procedure for "spam" ("many copies of the same message"), and relates the original and the re-typed comment thus at profile.

Hammond: my first comment to Stalin/out is not related with my picture and therefore appears at the subject only.

---

[1] To 'Stalin/out': "1934-1940 ultimately brought down" Hitler and Stalin

[2] Why do birds suddenly appear every time you are near, as clear as day?

[3] 'The Rule of Law in Ireland, end 2017' (December 19th 2017)

Robert Ewing – James May: "There it is, clear as day." Since profile no-longer relates the original second comment, it should be noted that it referred to legal professional "clear as day" reference to money, while this particular subject had arguable justification to refer to money, the subsequent subject did not, which is why I commented about reference to money to the subsequent subject and not to this subject: "There it is, clear as day." There is therefore no arguable justification for the deletion of the original second comment; and if that is not rectified I will cease involvement with this magazine.

Could anyone suppose pedestrians responsible for traffic-jams? Lay-litigants responsible for "clogging up" courts?[1] And fifteen hundred, not eleven hundred legal professionals – availability to right wrongs would reduce their number from fifteen to eleven. "You may feel that positions me on the level of an amoeba or vermin"; as I said:[2] "indecencies" – disrespectful as that was to my reference to "rats"; no serious discussion from Village; how could immense influence be defined as "amoeba or vermin"?

Robert Ewing – Profile again relates the original second comment;[3] thus note too that while we are in the hands of machines we can anticipate a system effectively dictated by probability; for example, disquis will not consult, rather must assume, concerning such statements as it labels "spam";[4] yet a legal statement, whether meant to be just or not, can be quoted as "case law", whether

---

[1]   Helen Collins' 'jam' was ignorance concerning the lists: "...brilliant..."

[2]   Received by the same subject writer: "particularly ...legal professional indecencies continue..."

[3]   And the original second comment continues not to appear at any subject

[4]   Reference to how disquis declares: "Detected as spam"

meant to be just or not; thus 'spam' by the State in such terms needs an inquiry procedure, rather than State response which, effectively, is the probability system of a machine, the standard 'probabilities' of which are exclusively anticipations of system performance; and since probability excludes the individual case, it is a convenient system to any machine, whether individually managed or technologically determined. In other words, our business and governing systems tend to be 'spam' based,[1] rather than 'spam' repellent; and at least one response to that injustice reads: "Detected as spam";[2] which is 'spam' ruling,[3] not the eradication of "spam"; which is "the virus" mentioned from the outset of my comments to Village; and we see and hear that "virus" every day in this jurisdiction with the business-like conduct of reporting national news – the news to report: the machine-like faces and voices of a media raised on spam.

---

[1] "Spam is flooding" /"overwhelming" /"a barrage" /"Most spam is commercial" /"most of the costs are paid for by the recipient or the carriers" /"spam is aimed" /"spam robs" /"spam subverts …systems"

[2] The commentator's allegation concluded as if alleging "spam": "the "endless" profession on behalf of Oleson's and the "endless" State."

[3] A regional newspaper subsequently related two responses to its: "A glimpse back into an Ireland we deny knowing"; the first ended: "Keep telling how it was/is", thus introduced: "Telling it as it was"; the second ("…power and control were centralised and still is", thus introduced: "Power is still centralised in Irish society"), misquoted the title (or was misquoted): "An Ireland we deny knowing." Denial of knowing thus, while relating that "we deny knowing"; "How they tried to keep you down if you weren't the son of a shopkeeper or businessman …putting everyone in a pidgeon hole." /"an Ireland that wanted to keep people down and in their place." "Power is still centralised"? Because "standing up for the vulnerable" challenges old ideas: the newspaper, supposed "a friend in court", would not however respond differently than "in the eighties", "as it was/is" spam; edited: "as it was", is media posture.

Bench marks

"I think most of the projects completed this year
have been of surprising value, especially to students
who have had no previous experience of a subject.
I think the real value lies not in the information
obtained but the deeper interest that they cultivate."
Robert Ewing, management student field project

"More than 30 years ago", began Supreme Court summary. "This is …more than thirty years ago", said Gore; and he lectured thus:

"Separating the truth from the fiction, and the accurate connections from the misunderstandings, is part of what you learn here."

The lecture I accepted more than thirty years ago was from a solicitor, and concerned the purported sale: "It cannot be done in Irish law." The lecture received by my co-defendant: "You wouldn't be in this mess if you hadn't taken the law into your own hands." However, anything can be lectured for Irish law "in this mess", because the legal profession have taken both the law and society into their own hands. "The trained official hates the rude, untrained public." State component 'misunderstanding' is the routine, not law.

"My proposal for world peace has therefore nothing to do with lecturing others, but instead centres on leading by example

– meaning that every individual must have direct procedural access to make their views known on matters that affect them at local government level ...it would ...remove countless misunderstandings between individuals and their [elected] authorities..."[1]

Subsequent to which, the Supreme Court lectured: "More than 30 years ago" /"must now be understood"; just as it had lied: "misunderstandings may arise"; "misunderstandings between individuals and their authorities"?

Subsequent to my pleading: "the conduct of the Gardai", Little Ship Street received a controversially deferential and inaccurate reply from them, as seems to be cultural relative to the routine of "lecturing others".

And as for citizen complaint process at local government level (including constituency office consultation process), it is routinely a culture of incident diary; no other procedure is involved; and, as with complaint concerning legal professionals generally, that suits the component culture, not least because the citizen is encouraged to rely on the State system and to trust it, and has had no training to 'corner' the errant component. Thus local government has an evasion culture, and citizen inexperience or ignorance is exploitable irrespective of whether they are complaining or not; procedures are based on a concept of component decency which simply invites the programming that complaints are incidents (unless they principally involve valid technicality); decency (or principle) is to be avoided; influence is the priority, such as instituting the litigation of 1987 as means to renew my father's dependency on solicitors sufficiently to undermine his property rights – a renewed consultation process

---

[1]   Robert Ewing to the Galway Advertiser (2006)

effectively dictated by the harasser's solicitor; and responding: 'incident', is cultural to obtaining influence, "as between solicitors", rather than responding relevantly, thus:

> "I knew Mr. ...K...y, ["but had not been in social or business contact with him for several years"] I had in fact acted in relation to family settlements etc for his father and mother several years before"

That referred to the question of "independent advice" and repeated the impression given to my father at the time; and was repeated to the Disciplinary Tribunal of the High Court:

> "I knew Mr. K...y and my firm had acted for him in the past as we would have for literally hundreds of families"

Not simply "in the past", for he "had acted for him" in his purchase of the lands involving the land-locked fields, and therefore subsequently had a conflict of interest "with Mr. Ewing"; thus:

> "Mr. Ewing was always aware that I had acted in the past for Mr. K...y. This was mentioned ...before Mr. K...y had been to my office with Mr. Ewing."

No legal diary existed to disprove that lie, because the complaint process itself is incident diary based; the solicitor and his client: "I knew Mr. K...y and my firm had acted for him in the past" /"for something that had happened."

"More than 30 years ago" /"must now be understood"; fraud "is part of what you learn" there.

Hitler's response to the Saarland vote for re-unification with Germany:

> "We are now certain that the time has come for appeasement and reconciliation." /"We want to assure the world of our deep desire to preserve the peace."

Re-unification meant less freedom for the Saarland; only Eden (an official interviewer of Hitler prior to the plebiscite) would not say so:

> "the Saar both before and during the plebiscite gave a glimpse of a supra-national salvation to a world which was imprisoning itself all the while more closely within the confines of the national state."[1]

Thus driven by position, rather than by performance, the State is "the nine-fifteen" of June 1942, and its relation to "Jack" is the nine-fifteen at Aberfan, or "this nettle, danger":

> "In all the circumstances it must be greatly regretted that the French government did not show more foresight and liquidate the Saar question by negotiation with Herr Hitler out of court, as he publically suggested, and in accordance with the advice of their ambassador in Berlin."[2]

"Hitler said ...the result would be a defeat for France and he wished to avoid this." "He thinks that they are stupid, ignorant,

---

[1]   Anthony Eden (1962)

[2]   Ambassador Eric Phibbs, January 1935

reckless – that they cannot tell their own interest – that they should have the leave of the office before they do anything. Protection is the natural inborn creed of every official…"; "the result of the Saar plebiscite has been to render Herr Hitler more independent and the omens less propitious for the success of any negotiations with this [coal mining] country."

"Chamberlain returned waving the treaty"?

Eden's "international statesman" had "failed" to make "the perfect inspirational speech"; "this should have been the time to strike out" with "fearless leadership", rather than with a "still cautious" and, therefore, less than "perfect" (indeed) "policy of appeasement" ("the further hesitations only served to improve Hitler's position").[1] "The truth is, that a skilled bureaucracy – a bureaucracy trained from early life to its special avocation – is though it boasts of an appearance of science, quite inconsistent with the true principles of the art of business."[2] And blame-game "science" (effectively, that 'livestock' will respond 'anxiously' or 'strongly', and their "rights of access to the courts" must concern land; for example: "the house is a very old large country farmhouse" – the "rat" said what a rat would think), has no principle:

> "The principal concern, therefore, of the plaintiff, ["the plaintiff's point of view of those proceedings" – "the proceedings concerning the land"] to which all of the allegations against the other defendants appear to be secondary, is to reopen the land dispute. This, as already stated…"

[1]   Samuel George (2008)
[2]   Walter Bagehot (1872)

My principal concern was the legal system, as would be the concern of truly legitimate custodianship of the dwelling. The Court did not mention its question to me concerning the land, to which I replied: "not really". It disregarded both that reply and my written pleading references to the dwelling, and thus lied: "appear" /"land dispute" (as would the High Court lie: apparently was "verbal"); to which I replied with proceedings against the State which referred to that lie; and to which the Court replied: "He now says that his concern in the 1996 [1999] set of proceedings was not really about the land..." (the Court thus related the words: "not really", but not "as already stated" by me, rather as: "but subsequently the Ewings"). The Court would have lied from the outset as it lied subsequently, only for its agenda to forward routine-like processing of its intended costs orders and those "already stated", rather than accept the controversy that the objective of the Circuit Court litigation was to halve the dwelling by way of money judgments and costs orders if the vendor refused "to settle". The Court could not therefore relate that "the 2 equity proceedings" were "the same", rather lie that the co-defendants had extended the dispute; and could not relate any significant reference to money (for example, the Court almost immediately lied: "sale ...for the sum of £45,000", rather than relate the agreed sum: "£35,000", and non-payment of the difference). And the High Court, by way of accepting the lie: "verbal agreement", would accept the harasser's 'costs' litigation 'now says', that the house need not be acquired (with deceitful reference to me such as began the victimization: "I think he probably wants some concession") – related by the Court as: "a concession", rather than relate that attempting to halve the dwelling led to the dispute, and that threatening acquisition

of the entirety of the dwelling had "already" been attempted
(the harasser claimed to me that he would own it if he paid the
"£45,000", in order to generate anxiety and negotiation). Such
was his litigation; and his application to the Land Commission
was also 'now says', rather than relate his attempt to dictate
halving of the dwelling.

"It was a retreat, but only in order to gain strength for a
further advance"?

"It was a concession"
"It was a retreat"
"It succeeded"

"It was a sign of Lenin's genius"[1] even, to "try, try, try again"?
Clearly exile in England had advanced his politics:

"Upton's on a hill" / "Hang (and I mean hang so that the
people can see) not less than 100 known kulaks, rich
men, bloodsuckers."

"Hammerton's in a hole" / "Publish their names."

"Winwick blows the bellows" / "Take all their grain away
from them."

"And Thurning provides the coal." / "Identify hostages
as we described in our telegram yesterday. Do this so
that for hundreds of miles around the people can see,
tremble, know and cry: they are killing and will go on
killing the blood-sucking kulaks.

---

[1] Stephen King-Hall (1961)

Cable that you have received this and carried out your instructions. Yours, Lenin

P.S. Find tougher people"

"P.S. Find tougher people"? Exile in Geneva had influenced him too; only he concluded thus as insufficiently tough to claim his future? Yet it was another genius who was exiled:

"Czechoslovakia was no lost German province but an independent nation, allied to Britain, France and the Soviet Union." /"Britain and France gave way..."[1] /"Chamberlain returned waving the treaty..."

"Find tougher people"?

"Czechoslovakia was tough", and "Russia stood ready to back concerted action against Germany..."[2]

Britain had *no* treaty with Czechoslovakia, or with France ("By 1937 French foreign policy lay in ruins"),[3] or with the Soviet Union: "one cannot in all circumstances undertake" agreement with Russia and disagreement with France.

"France gave way"; and Chamberlain, waving from the doorway of the plane for Germany, would ultimately display and relate the peoples declaration that "once again there was to be no concerted action against Germany"; subsequent to which Germany would obtain a treaty with "ready" Russia, dividing Poland between them, and the war led to more waving, only

---

[1]   The World at War (1974)

[2]   USA service information film 2

[3]   Alfred Cobban (1965)

as follows: "the British weren't ready for it."[1] An historical confusion thus evident concerning a war initially involving Poland, now assumed to be a war initially involving Norway: April 1940 confused with September 1939, by way of reference to the so-called "phony war" (September 1939 to April 1940), and the equivalent phony peace which preceded it (as Chamberlain put it, Hitler's termination of Czechoslovak independence was "a mockery" of peace); Chamberlain personified as the indifferent ("a quarrel in a far-away country between people of whom we know nothing"), or unreal ("I recommend you to go home and sleep quietly in your beds"), administrator; indeed, such as was only "at last beginning to understand dimly something of the situation" that "French foreign policy lay in ruins", not in Rouen.

However, "I think the real value lies not in the information obtained but the deeper interest": the infallibility of society versus "a policy of appeasement" – supposed example of the fallibility (and even duplicity) of institutions?

> "Churchill knew that this was a time not for reason, but for faith…"[2]

The infallibility of society, on the one hand, and on the other hand: the fallible society tendency to respect belief (or "faith") first – consideration (or action) second? Otherwise: "The battle of Britain": defiance or defence?

"Our motto is not defiance, and, mark my words, it is not, either, deference. It is defence, and we confidently count on the response of the nation to make that defence invincible."

---

[1] The World at War (1974)
[2] 'Heritage of Britain' by Reader's Digest Assoc. Ltd

"I [Chamberlain] cannot take Russia very seriously as an aggressive force, though no doubt formidable if attacked in her own country"; I initially believed in judge availability as much as I believed in solicitor non-availability, as concerned challenging the harassment; but the legal professional culture is one of report, not law; as Supreme Court judge Niall McCarthy effectively related that culture: "uncritical".

"Understand that solicitors engage in legitimate deceit (such as bluffing client readiness to institute proceedings)." /""We need" procedural safeguards; eliminate the 'decent chaps' equation ...target the dated system: ...garbage ...provides rats with both cover and nourishment".

"You may feel that positions me on the level of an amoeba or vermin"? Village readers were thus invited to assume that the subject writer was unaware of any attempt to begin a debate concerning the legal system, and thus assume as an academic concluded: "human society"; acceptance of which is a "descending into anarchy" (such as alleged against the co-defendants: "a terrible problem" which would ultimately invite "serious trouble"). Humanity invites debate, not lecturing, but debate is alien to the State, which seeks agreement "as between Solicitors" – as between colleagues, and not as between different parts of society: "The learned High Court Judge concluded his judgment, as he had started it ...rather than with any evaluation of the matters which are clearly of concern to the plaintiff and are the subject of his complaint, but which are..."; "thus did I receive statement of moral issues in case conclusions", for while "the profession clearly prefers to stay away from moral questions", alleging complainant allegation as stating: "amoeba or vermin", is to allege incident, and thereby avoid the 'tougher muses', such as: "no reaction from solicitors" /'no threat of proceedings, just the litigation itself over a year later' (May 1986 to June 1987). Moral issues: my involvement with the harasser began aged rather closer to fourteen than fifteen, as evidence, including a Christmas card, relates. I was nineteen when he persuaded my father to tell me that he had purchased the land (the same lie that the High Court and Supreme Court would tell "the Irish people themselves", rather that relate that the dwelling was transferred and the harassment monies had resumed – the harasser's proposed price for the land having been agreed: £35,000). He would generate anxiousness for negotiation purposes by saying to me that he could own the entirety of the lands if he paid the fictional contract sum of "£45,000"; however he would ultimately propose to pay "£55,000" (the land had been valued at "£50,000", and the dwelling at "£25,000"); subsequent to which I obtained independent advice that the non-payment of "£45,000" meant no sale, which guaranteed ending the harassment (as indisputably that sum had not been paid), and thereby resolving the access controversy; only the harasser and the legal profession would not respect the various relevant property rights unless they were solicitor supported, just as the State itself accepts reports as between components (a routine of which is to state: "resolve", or "helpful", or "best interest" - "best interests"), rather than encourage report as between the public and the State: the first Supreme Court would only state: "the sum of £45,000", and "deed of transfer dated the 2nd day of January 1983" (the written pleading clarified: "a Sunday"); and the second Court would perpetuate its non-mention of the re-transfer by way of relating the sum of "£35,000", and, consequently, did not relate the sum of "£45,000". Discovery related that the vendor proposed

"£40,000" for the land, but the legal profession would process that sum as reply not to "£35,000" but "£30,000" – yet another false sum to convenience the harassment, just as a solicitor of the jurisdiction conceded privately: 'The side telling the most lies usually wins.'

"It's the same the whole world over" /"Equality, Rights and Justice Guarantees:

- Fulfilment of fundamental and inalienable social, economic, cultural, civil, political and environmental rights.
- Equality between women and men.
- Protection from sexual violence and exploitation, and caring support to allow for control of fertility and family planning.
- Equality for all people and diverse groups in our society, respectful of diversity of age, disability, gender, religion, ethnic identity - including membership of the Traveller community, sexual orientation, marital status, family status, or socio-economic status.
- Protection from institutional abuses, isolation, segregation, discrimination and violence, together with equal treatment before the law.
- Equitable distribution of income so as to ensure a guaranteed adequate minimum income for all, whether in paid employment or not, which is sufficient to live life in comfort and with dignity, achieving a socially acceptable ratio between maximum and minimum incomes."

"It's the poor what gets the blame" /"Participatory, Accountability and Inclusive Democracy Guarantees:

- Pluralist, participatory, diverse, gender-balanced and accountable democracy, with strong local government and inclusive systems of decision-making, which listens to all voices and reflects collective opinion, celebrating diversity of opinion and dissent.
- Public participation in policy-making, including for those experiencing poverty, inequality, and social exclusion; and a constructive say in decisions.
- Vibrant civil society with effective community and environmental organisations, trade unions, community-culture groups and cooperative enterprises which, through collective effort, build strong communities which are flourishing places of caring, sharing and well-being.
- Safe and legal avenues to enter Ireland for those from outside Europe who are in need of our protection and an assurance of welcome, integration and empowerment for migrants and refugees.
- Opportunities to express creativity and participate in and celebrate our social and cultural heritage as well as the traditions of other cultures in our society."

"It's the rich what gets the gravy" /"Sustainable Environment and Vibrant Economy Guarantees:

- Environment that is protected, renewed, and made available for future generations; is freed from the use of

fossil fuel; promotes recycling; and values and protects
its biodiversity.
- Vibrant economy that serves the needs of society,
  provides sustainable jobs and respects environmental
  limits: an economy that promotes the development
  of cooperative enterprises and that organises the
  production, distribution and consumption of goods
  and resources in an egalitarian and environmentally
  sustainable way.
- Banking and financial system that is strongly regulated
  and prohibits excessive speculation and rewards.
- Progressive, just and equitable taxation system that
  balances taxes on labour, wealth, corporate profits,
  financial transactions and resources, that fosters equality
  and that enables long-term sustained investment in our
  public infrastructure and services.
- Decent, properly rewarded, accessible and non-
  exploitative work, job security, workers' rights, equal
  pay for men and women and a good work-life balance."

"Ain't it all a bloomin' shame." /"High Quality of Life based on
Solidarity Guarantees:

- Effective, efficient, transparent and adequately funded
  public services available to all irrespective of income
  and, in particular, effective, efficient and universally
  accessible public health services, social services,
  education, early childhood care and education, and
  transport services.
- Secular education system that empowers young people
  to develop as active citizens, giving them practical

experience of civic life, informing them of the rights they enjoy and should respect, and supporting them to participate in shaping their future.

- Affordable, high quality, warm and energy-efficient homes, both public and private, available to all as a right.
- Well-being of all children who will be cherished and loved equally and will have access to shelter, food, education and other services necessary for their happiness and development; no child will grow up in an institutional environment and no child will be subjected to sexual exploitation.
- Recognition of and support for the contribution of care-work and voluntary activity to society."[1]

"Ain't it all a bloomin' shame"? All a polling card and a tax form: "What are you [William Ewing] keeping that old man ["the surviving spouse"] alive for, wouldn't you be better off if he was dead." Hearing he had died (a termination of his remaining rights), the harasser "immediately" obtained a meeting involving his workman (a member of his household), who "simply spent the evening staring at me, and listening intently to what was being said"; which began: "I can't go on like this anymore – I don't wish to graze the land any longer. I can't do anything with it." My father thus proposed sale of the "River" field, and the corner of another field between it and the public road; which was agreed, as was the routine stealth.

"I couldn't understand why [the workman] was there and I tried to ignore him." And the workman would be routinely

---

[1] Claiming Our Future centenary proclamation (2016)

involved during the dispute, but only prior to the litigation: "If [the workman] ...comes up, and drags you out of the house, and beats you up, it won't have anything to do with me." Such were the 'loans' convenience based, as was the involvement of lawyers; senior counsel "banging the table"? "I can't go on like this anymore..."

Meanwhile, however, my father had met a retired judge and referred to the movie: "The field", in order to relate his concept of a book about the dispute: "The *three* fields", while unaware that Marchington had, or would have, a sign of village genius: "Threefields". Historical legacies, indeed:

> "The Three Fields" /"The barrister mentioned the [tenant's temporary] gate (new gate) across the laneway. ["the laneway" access was ordered a life-time previous as rights available to family members only] The judge said that how could the Ewings be penalized for this, when the laneway was on the portion of land that Mr. K...y claimed did not belong to him. The barrister replied that the laneway was for Mr. K...y to get into three fields that he owned, before the sale from Mr. Ewing. The judge held up the map with the yellow shading showing the laneway ...did not connect with the three fields ... The judge said that if this was a family arrangement [effectively reference to the court order] he did not see how Mr. K...y could claim a right of way, there being no right of way registered."

> "The Three Pigeons" /"Mr. Ewing asked Mr. K...y how he would get into his three fields [no longer land-locked if he had bought the Ewing land – to which there was

considerable road-frontage and already a new gate]
without the use of the laneway? Mr. K...y did not reply.
[He could not relate that if he had bought the Ewing land,
the laneway was basically a lever by which to obtain
more of the property] Judge Cassidy intervened and said
"By helicopter", to which Mr. K...y replied: "Exactly."

Surely Mr. K...y [the registered owner of the lands]
should have said 'through the land that I bought from
Mr. Ewing'..."

"By helicopter"? Control of the discussion consistent with State
component inclinations generally and the lecturer's conclusion:
"that most astounding and troublesome of all phenomena, human
society". Indeed, "no control", as my co-defendant alleged; our
natural concerns negated by clever labeling: "you [who would
give blood] are a co executor" /"you [who wrote at college
that helicopters would be the ambulances of the future] are the
owner" /"you [who gave driving-school lessons and acquired the
school] are now changing your instructions". "The *three* fields",
indeed:

> The legal profession generally only has one case
> Every case is treated the same
> And every word they use is convenient to them.

"TEA"? Indeed, tax it, rather than its prey: human society. Find
the debate, rather than conclude: "we're much better"; "you
are"? Indeed, "we're" not:

> "my second comment ...could not be found"

I therefore repeated the comment to the recently posted published subject, but that too disappeared, and subsequently the following comment happened to appear there:

> "What a brilliant insight into one of the most corrupt little islands in the world. We should be made to start again."

Prior to my reading which, "Bench marks" concluded:

> "TEA"? Tax it, rather than its prey: human society. Find the debate, rather than conclude: "and we're much better"; "you are"? Indeed, "we're" not.

"Indeed you are" much better? "All God's children" ("The Three Pigeons" indeed): "Or are you?"

"The barrister replied that the laneway was for Mr. K...y to get into three fields that he owned, before the sale from Mr. Ewing." The harasser's reply to my father subsequent to the Circuit Court litigation: "It's convenient." Indeed, a life of convenience to oneself: "it was not my instruction that Robert should not be involved in the case" /"the legal team did not seem to want my son by my side, and indeed I was warned, that ... Robert was involved." 'Ain't it all the son', was the agreement between the various solicitors; they too were "using me as an excuse to change direction." I was escorting the vulnerable to school, so-to-speak, only the school itself contained the equivalent danger of responding to either "legal" or "natural" inconvenience as incident - the lecturers could not be led, because they had but one communication: "start again", "and we're much better", as is the standard education theory for which even Bagehot was optimistic:

> "A new Constitution does not produce its full effect as long as all its subjects were reared under an old Constitution, as long as its statesmen were trained by that old Constitution."

Indeed, find the debate, rather than follow elitist "closed-shop", such as dictates that an agreement drawn-up by a lawyer cannot be challenged, *except by another lawyer* - "we" thus divided by "We"; family and home, like Poland, divided by dictatorship 'business as usual'; even assistance between members of a family succession negated, rather than allow "natural" result to 'business as usual' mistakes.

"Of course this Court is sympathetic to any litigant" not relying on the "professional lawyer"; lay-litigants "may be mistaken", but professionals understand the State's "declaration of aims"? I replied: "the document ...has but one aim..." "Of course Mr. Robert Ewing..."

"Find the debate", "rather than sticking empty labels."

"The ["gallant"] Duke of Brunswick received the mortal shot when ...lighting a fresh cigar at the pipe of one" Stanley Baldwin? Thus "Chamberlain returned waving" matches?

"Most of this is sales talk by academics anxious to justify their existence."[1] The gallant Duke of Wellington: "I think the best thing you can do is to go to bed."

"Really I have no need to defend my visits to Germany last autumn, for what was the alternative?"

---

[1]   A.J.P. Taylor (1977)

He too generally only had one case? "But I had another purpose, too, in going to Munich."

In other words, human beings have more than one work advantage over machines. For example: the mobilisation of the Czar's army was unstoppable once begun – effectively a mechanism which could only "provide its full effect"; just as State component positions and procedures tend to perpetuate themselves irrespective of their effectiveness and the State "generally only has one case"; therefore it is not necessarily true that either rearing or training will evolve as Bagehot anticipated, and therefore it is not necessarily the case that the State official is sufficiently humanised to "strike out" as would "fearless leadership" to maintain "the dignity and freedom of the individual" – that would take a Chamberlain to prepare, as Churchill advised: "You & I can command everything if we work together."

"Meanwhile, however, the Italian dictator, looking for a little cheap glory, had decided on Abysinnia";[1] that I would deny that "the Gardai and legal profession" "can claim moral or intellectual distinction"; and would blame "Irish people themselves", rather than "the ruling classes" or State; and would ask a court to "direct the government"?

"Hitler was looking for someone to blame", said Andrew Marr, rather than conclude: 'lecture'.

Thus had the German dictator, looking for a little cheap glory (someone to lecture), "missed the bus"; for he generally only had one direction, and his foreign minister thus flew to Moscow and returned 'waving the treaty', yet oblivious that Hitler was blaming the German people themselves, and would

---

[1]   Alfred Cobban (1965)

only really hurry toward Moscow after he began to also blame himself for missed buses.

The "Polish Corridor" - the "stupid, ignorant, reckless" division of Germany, on the one hand, and, on the other hand: "I [Chamberlain] doubt if any solution, short of war, is practicable at present"? Hitler and Stalin would agree for half each, just as Czechoslovakia was initially halved between conflicting interests; but Chamberlain would "command everything" of Poland, and would indeed resolve the "stupid, ignorant, reckless" division, rather than allow a "stupid, ignorant, reckless" descent into the "stupid, ignorant, reckless" cycle of European "uncertainty" – "that atmosphere of surprise and alarm from which Europe has suffered", and which had but one advantage "for people who believe in liberty" ("like President Roosevelt"): "the possibility of such a departure as we are now contemplating", rather than "confine ourselves to a single case which, after all, might not be the case in point" ("a ...case" of "stupid, ignorant, reckless" division, on the one hand, and "the case" of "a demand to dominate one by one other nations without limits to where that might go", on the other hand). "It might be a case of..." "stupid, ignorant, reckless" division. Indeed, that was not *the* case, which was "a demand to dominate", "which wins nothing, cures nothing, ends nothing"; "multiplied by a thousand" corridors; "one case" machines "multiplied by a thousand"; the reply to which was, indeed: "I doubt if any solution, short of war, is practicable at present."

"You & I", indeed, "and we're much better", indeed, "if we work together."

The Times: "Worcester could be Wooster" – "Wooster Sauce"? Just as "sauce" could be "source" and "School Lane" could be "India Street"?

"Justice Arun Mishra said it would be more humane for governments to murder their own citizens and grant them a quick death" thereby.[1] That concisely contradicted "claim that the legal profession and I have absolutely nothing in common". Thus "the most sense in the most appropriate direction" could be "the bench" - just as "Arun" could be "Kyle" to Hugh Tomlinson today, otherwise: "You & I".

"Mr Ewing has reviewed the matter, he has pointed out that this appeal ["work together"] was necessary to obtain certainty. He expressed his appreciation for the judgment of ["India's Supreme"] ...Court because it did as he said provide certainty and finality in the matter": the whole history of legal professional obstruction to "the Ewings" was a consequence of legal professional culture not to judge one another, a consequence of which was that Irish Supreme court lie and the conduct of the future judge who Robert Ewing judged on the 17th January 1985, effectively the "signal duty" of judging the cultures involved. And thus if State components are not prepared to accept good judgment by way of that "vague public mind", the public should ask as Mishra did: "Why should people suffer this?" The real judge ("the supremo") supposedly attempted to obstruct performance of a sale; judged his case "rightly dismissed"; and instituted claim that the dismissal was wrong; thus "know ... instructions meant nothing" – "public policy" meant nothing; "public relations" is the art of categorization and means more to State components than hearing: "You wouldn't be in this mess if you hadn't taken the law into your own hands" – partisan counsel against attempt to obtain legal process for "the law". "The public

---

[1] Interpretations by The Times (27 November 2019) subsequent to the original conclusion of this chapter published on page 183: "work together."

has a right to know" and to judge: "The vague public mind" could be 'the art of citizen survival'; yet what do we hear of that art? Nothing, because partisanship is the dominant culture, not citizen survival, thus with ice-cold hostility: "Get out of my office!"

"The public has the right to know:" "Get explosives ...kill them [the 'Kyle parish' victims] in one go. Why should people suffer this?" The public can know: "Why not" /"call to bring down the virus", could be: "Why not call to bring down the virus?" In other words, the first words of The Times report: "India's Supreme Court has said it would be "better"..." thus could be "much better" as "Preambulary introduction..." - "Bench marks" could be "the true principles of the art of business", which are the only justifications, the true generic qualifications, for office; "grant them" a long life.

Friends of the road

"Any time you want to run over a song or anthem let
me know & we can fix a half-hour or so. Meantime
go forward with confidence. God rest you merry –
let *nothing* you dismay!"
Frank Cowle to William Ewing, November 1958

Bagehot's "traditionary Irishman on his visit to Donnybrook
Fair, 'Wherever you see a head hit it.'" The Fair must have had
a "crown green".

The Fourth man (the captain) of the historic indoor Fours of
the republican jurisdiction could usually redirect trouble with a
fast wood, and therefore it was my opinion, as Third man, not to
interrupt him once he began preparing his shot.

However, as the Four was compiled of two clubs, it could
not continue for lawn-green club matches; and consequently I
was First or Second to that captain, and Third interrupted him
preparing his final "wood", which was a "firing" shot, to a
'barn-door' of about seven "shots" which threatened to leave us
far behind, more than half-way through the match; "somewhat
slow progress" - "will keep you informed of progress, if any."
The "fire" only scorched a distant side of the 'barn', costing us
our 'turf-accountancy' credit for the remainder of that Third and
Fourth "Paddy's" day.

A few months later I advised my co-defendant concerning his first meeting with senior counsel: "You have to get what *you* want from this meeting, not what *they* want; or we shall never see the light of day."

By that time I was the first indoor singles champion (of champions) of the jurisdiction, and that season had been "Lead" to a former international. I subsequently visited my mother's home-town for the first time, and wrote to the Clare Champion about the legal system and Irish society (most prescient or intuitive relative to a reported policing controversy and controversies at Ennis courthouse): "a culture of diary and interest, rather than de Valera standing on O'Connell's shoulders as if the phoenix rising from the ashes of a meeting that never takes place." A culture "to bring people together, contrary to what was being inferred" – alleging: "raising cane", as began in December 1984 and was related annually to October 1988, as noted by my father: "a smokescreen".

He ("a very quiet, shy almost, man with a fine baritone voice")[1] was that type of person: diary and interest.

"This man ['hooked on classics': "Let the courts decide" /"It's K…n M…s' case"] has had headaches much of the time over the last few months which appear to be worse when dealing with [as the least relevant professional would conclude:] the stress of his court case. He has also developed high blood pressure and this I think could also be related to stress. I therefore feel that the court case in which he is involved is having a considerable effect on his health." The progress was not as a professional would report it, or as he had reported: "everything going our way, but slowly"; it was as he subsequently reported to St Brendan's

---

[1]   Arthur Moyse to Robert Ewing (1999)

church: "somewhat slow progress towards the court room" /"will keep you informed of progress, if any." Matches lent and not returned? Perhaps the question was less about a pipe and a cigar, and more about whether the people control the State, or the State control the people?

> District Court judge: "Have you ever heard of a guillotine?"
> "Yes, off with the head."
> "Once that was used, that was the end of the matter. I'll give you limited sympathy …but you are walking toward a guillotine."

My "Human Societies" has a name in it: "J.A. Kyle." "Be careful lad, To keep out of the lawyer's claw".[1] I had been careful, but only since the negotiations accepted by me while unaware of the various allegations against me, and aware of the unavailability of solicitors; since we did not challenge the right of way claim, and I was unaware of the "guarantee" which had been sought a year before ("Needs guarantee of this…"), it seemed to me that the negotiations had increased my father's vulnerability to solicitors dictating acceptance of the harassment, even while the non-challenge was part of our attempt to resolve the various issues. Thus I attempted to safeguard my father from the consequences of accepting the negotiations; but as is "the lawyer's claw", that attempt was misrepresented as our having taken the law into our "own hands".

"It is important to stress", and "the lawyer's claw" routinely does that, as at my father's first consultation with the solicitor

---

[1]   The Cottage Well Thatched With Straw

on returning to live in Ireland: "You have no responsibility for that man ["the surviving spouse"] what-so-ever"; just as the independent solicitor involved would change his tune concerning my father [inadvertently thereby alerting me to the letter marked 'personal' which lied: "Of course Mr. Robert Ewing..." /"we will have to inform Mr. ...K...y" – claiming valid "responsibility for that man"]: "Don't bring that man into me."[1] The "one case" each time, rather than attempt to resolve the various issues; the dispute allegedly generated by "the type of person Robert was", only "Mr. K...y was the person", and was reported as such (concerning "the surviving spouse", prior to my father returning to Ireland), by the falsely accused "one local man". The "one case" claim of "the type of person" who chooses to live in rural Ireland: "wanted ...for questioning in connection with wounding live-stock". And "they could not locate him"? Co-defendant junior counsel "could not be found" at the courthouse (lied the second solicitors), but would be questioned by my co-defendant (exactly as I had advised), and replied with "woe", just as I had warned as lay-solicitor or counsel with "responsibility for that man".

"I'll give you limited sympathy ...but you are..." "You are only a blow-in." "Have you ever heard of a guillotine?"

"This man" was very weak at our last meeting; he phoned from the coach-station and intended to remain there, but I managed to persuade him to move to the front steps of the Custom House (adjacent to the coach-station) where we could sit and discuss our litigation plans in an appropriate environment (and I was unaware that the warship moored nearby the previous

---

[1]   Robert Tombs (2017): "response ...boorish, insulting and threatening"

day had departed).[1] We had already expressed our good-byes to one-another; yet it was strange that when he stood up from the steps he turned to pick up his bag, rather than postpone 'any other business' for his usual eye-contact greeting; and, remarkably, as he slowly reached for his bag he appeared to me as if frozen in Time, as if part of an historic photograph: part of History.

I walked the quayside footpath at a pace, and once he thought I surely saw him, he stood up with the intention of crossing the road to a seat-bench, and I therefore continued along the quayside, and we crossed the road at the bridge and sat on one of the nearby quayside benches, he closest to the bridge; and I gave him an art book (coloured by a number of his children), the last page of which also had a word: "Pax", which, as I expressed to him, appeared as if printed across the dwelling-side of his external yard-gate; he responded slowly: "Can I have this?" I replied: "I brought it for you."

We discussed his meeting of the previous day, which was with the former lay-litigant, Barbara Hyland (who was dying and had been the election candidate who meant to "oblige the government to appoint a legal ombudsman"); and I prodded the bench between us several times while declaring: "You have a unique case in Irish legal history." And more slowly: "You have a unique case in Irish legal history."

He had brought his High Court procedural guidebook with him, and therefore had a book to pass to me, which he brought forth from his bag with great heart despite the extraordinary look of departure in his eyes; and as we reached the coach-station, his strength much recovered, he said, referring to our plan to

---

[1] We had visited his brother's memorial (the merchant navy memorial) a few years previously, which is almost adjacent to the "Belfast".

meet a few days later: "And I will look forward to seeing you in Belfast on Thursday." We parted inside the coach-station where he had spoken his last words to any member of his family: "And now, Robert, I am going home." I last saw him as we walked to our respective coaches (his parked at an angle to the controller's position meant that he re-appeared); he walking beside his with his head down. His coach journey would pass his first home, where he was born and his mother died; and he died at her first home and birth-place, and the corpse was driven away at the said yard-gate. A former choir member recalled him singing the line ending: "a great light"; and my father had turned, meaning to reply to my last words to him, his hand raised as at his passing two days later (reacting from his sleep); and there was great light in his eyes; I had turned to him and said: "We're *going to* win."

The year previous he brought me an old book showing a sketch of Hougoumont[1] (part of the battlefield at Waterloo) on its title-page; and the year previous expressed to me that I should write the history of the dispute (once the attempt to obtain justice from the courts concluded); but such was the conclusion of our intended litigation, and of my experience of "Human Rights" and the government, that I had also to write to the president about the disregard for hearings, thus:

> "Every now and then a feeling of almost irresistible nausea and revulsion comes over me at the thought of all the drudgery, the humiliation, the meaness and pettiness of that life, and of the hopeless impossibility of getting things done."
>
> *Neville Chamberlain*

---

[1]   "We had the wood behind ...we could have made good the wood"

1, Irish government informed December 1989: negligence panel solicitor "not taking any notice" of allegations concerning then judge of the District Court (solicitor relation to William Ewing), my concern being that there would not be evidence of obstruction of justice by [co-defendant] counsel at hearing by which such obstruction could be litigated.

2, Various then unknown factors produced the necessary evidence: the correspondence from solicitors over the long period of what William Ewing described as "the delaying tactics of the legal profession" (1995); our written communications showing expectation that counsel would represent us both at hearing (the orders relate that he did not); Circuit Court judge would not conclude hearing at which we had no lawyers (1990), and William Ewing wrote a record of that hearing for solicitors; and applications to the disciplinary tribunal of the High Court caused hearing record from 'the other side' to pass into our possession, concerning the Circuit Court hearing which did conclude (1996), therefore the obstruction of justice by counsel in 1996 is apparent to anyone.

3, Since neither the High Court nor the Supreme Court take any notice of allegations of obstruction of justice by counsels, the concern that caused report to the government had no relation to the actual circumstances – the courts would not accept the allegations, and therefore would not accept the evidence that hearing process was breached.

4, Their obstruction of justice was apparent to anyone (2000/2001), and this caused litigation against the State itself, which necessarily caused the difficult situation of the High Court having to consider allegations against the Supreme Court; both courts continued as before (2008/2013) to obstruct process, with the Supreme Court again misquoting pleading to suit the system breach; yet again: "not taking any notice".

5, The report of December 1989 partly related that the Law Society did not appear concerned about the legal system breach alleged. The Society's response appears typical of the subsequent responses from State components; no part of the State system appears concerned about any allegation of system breach; procedural rules are supposed to ensure against attempted breach, only they 'serve' to guarantee the breach already perpetrated. In other words, no part of the State system appears to be concerned about breach of the legal system, and the legal profession is therefore practically invited to do whatever it likes with the system, thereby inviting the negligence alleged by William Ewing.

The negligence panel solicitors noted: "He said that he felt things were moving in a positive direction now and if a Judge put him out on the side of the road well he would accept that but at least the whole matter would have been adjudicated upon by an independent party."

"Judge put him out on the side of the road well" that might explain why some people end up there, because their belief-system is as the colleges and media would have it, and not as the money-culture is inclined to reward. "He doesn't know the first thing" about business, complained the same solicitor to me; and that too, whatever it meant, vindicated my initiatives. Yet neither his involvement nor mine was of the experienced professional; and Chamberlain, for example, was not a legal professional, and could appear not to know the first thing about lawyers:

> "I trust that our action, begun but not concluded, will prove to be the turning point not towards war, which wins nothing, cures nothing, ends nothing, but towards a more wholesome era when reason will take the place of force and threats will give way for cool and well-marshalled arguments."

"The outstanding qualities of Mr. Chamberlain are courage, consistency and logic."[1] "I appreciated your observations ...and agree with you. It's good to know we have a friend in Bedford":[2]

> "During the early days of his premiership one thing struck me [Lawrence Burgis] most forceably and that was the courtesy and deference with which Churchill treated Neville Chamberlain."[3]

'Well, at all events this train belongs to me', said Alan Peglar; to which the board of trade bureaucracy replied as if his points pleaded revolutionary Boston.[4]

---

[1] Duff Cooper, November 1938

[2] The Ford administration to John Donelan (1974)

[3] This was not "general appeasement" but alliance presumed to most advantage the general war effort

[4] Flying Scotsman USA

The 'wheel-tappers and shunters social' utopia on British trains: 'Well, at all events these verbal platform security messages will not be verbal on the trains themselves'? To which the board of spam (or 'community wreckers anonymous') presumably would reply: 'Well, at all events this train belongs to spam'.

"Robert [aged eleven] is to be congratulated". And if the conclusion: "forceably", had any great significance it is that Kingsley Wood's advice to Churchill to 'free-wheel' his way through the succession meeting with Chamberlain and Halifax, derived from a traditionary alliance between Chamberlain and Churchill, one of the consequences of which had been that Churchill received the principal public credit for State debt principally owed to Chamberlain. As Churchill conceded to him, concerning Hitler's proposed conference at Munich: "You were very lucky."

"Being civilised [or relatively ignorant] becomes a crucial sign of weakness or opportunity to the unscrupulous and the cynical."[1] Hence "a cornered rat" ("irked" despite "More than 30 years" experience, by my "thoroughly professional manner" concerning his lie: "40"). "Every day of the week we" disregard and interrupt, "and if everybody who thought that they had" the "will"… "Every day of the week", stealth towards "force and threats"; against which, for example, was "the office" in India Street: "if he gets the opportunity, he ought to do well on the Technical side"; and he did:

> "When asked about the £13,500 amount which shows on his [the harasser's] list of payments for sale, dated March '83, he seemed at a loss to explain the two payments

---

[1]   Village, April 2017

being the same, but the dates [December 1982 and March] somewhat apart."

Subsequent Circuit Court pleading against the co-defendants: "about the turn of the last Century"; consistent with which was denial that both co-defendants had lawyers involved and subsequent to which the Supreme Court referred to the two different sale sums "somewhat apart" (in 2001 referring to the £45,000, and in 2013 the £35,000); every relationship "somewhat apart"; the Court would not relate that it received a document which stated (as the Limerick Leader newspaper had stated of my father, one of the singing and acting "four dudes"), for example:

> "I say, as a matter of supreme importance, that myself and my father's true characters and place in Irish – and perhaps even in INTERNATIONAL society, have been denied to us by the [relevant High Court] defendants in this Case. I, like my father before me, and as I was when he was alive, DO NOT EXIST in this State."

I cast his ashes across the lawn from an erne wrapped in his European Union flag, and then placed the flag, together with its 'remains of the day', in the erne, where it is to this day.

His father's last words to him seem to have been prescient or intuitive (he gestured as if a case was beneath his bed but nothing was there): "Get the case." /"The case." My father's reference to me at the conclusion of his first meeting with senior counsel: "The most important person isn't here." I spoke my sentiments at the time of advising the dispute, and almost quarter of a century later Fintan O'Toole (regarded by Village as Ireland's leading intellectual), wrote the same words as title to his book meant to begin debate concerning cultural non-performance of the State: "Enough is enough".

"A reliable duty assistant", aged fifteen; and duty called at eleven: "Robert [aged eleven] has shown less interest of late. His original enthusiasm is lacking." I immediately wrote thereat: "Complete rubbish"; and the subsequent term report from the same teacher concerning the same subject said: "Excellent work – he always shows interest & enthusiasm."

"Robert is maintaining the standards".

"Yes, off with the head", is the Third, just as 'off with the claw' is the guillotine, so-to-speak, which "isn't here."

Thus if the man living on a pavement is a Well for "acute cultural analysis", the money-culture and revenue system will not purposefully offer his examiner "a lift"; it will say he is "a dunce" at loggerheads with people not properly understood by him. And thus will one find the minister at the Land Registry, just as one will find the "rat" ("and we are") at the Law Society, "checking on the Law Society rulings in relation to the matter." A culture of social climbing by way of "two faces";[1] one "may" (to appear interested), the other "must" (to appear authority): "it may be a case of... (finished in Latin)" /"it must now be understood".

"Yes, off with the head." And off with the "claw".

Judge Cassidy did not translate his Latin, just as a Supreme Court principal interrupted on the side of the negligence panel solicitors and had "absolutely no explanation whatsoever for taking such a view"; just as had been related to the Irish Times by the electioneer: "whenever complaints are not dealt with to the

---

[1]   Writers and Jay and Lynn

complainant's satisfaction, the society fails to provide them any, or any adequate explanation"; "dissatisfied with the judgment", stated the High Court, as would statement of complaint be from either "the society" or the minister, or as is a common litigant reaction to judgments; the probability relation: assume the latter, rather than assume professional negligence or fraud.

Thus can the origins of the dispute be summed up as the electioneer alleged: "and protect our own"; "*and* protect our own". For example, the Supreme Court would disregard my pleading and quote a number of the High Court's statements to the effect that I had failed to provide any, or any adequate explanation, for the litigation; and lied that I confirmed the technical validity of the Court's purported quotation of my pleading; "protect our own"; suggest the succession to be 'yesterdays news', "as I have already said", and, as such, suggest that its legal trial was consistent with claiming "centuries of trial" and/or with supposing neglect to understand the legal profession, if only to appear consistent with the declared interests of the State, and if only routine – the legal profession has the least interest in contemporary legal cases.

"Robert [aged fifteen] sets very high standards for himself." Twenty-six counties, "as I have written previously, does not as a state conform to the rule of law."[1]

The plaintiff's senior counsel had his head in his hands as I spoke to judge Cassidy, and co-defendant senior counsel would be "banging the table to show his displeasure"; indeed, as is "likely to overlook the end in the means; it will fail from narrowness of mind; it will be eager in seeming to do; it will be idle in real doing." The profession may seem as if it is going

---

[1]   Village, March 2017

out of its way, but it goes nowhere, such is its way, as I have observed; State components generally know that complaints generally concern decency – a consideration for moral issues which generally will lead nowhere, and, indeed, "to nothing…"

Indeed, "see a head" in hands, "hit it": the purchaser had tried very hard to bring my parents back together, as further means to influence my father. "Mr. K…y shook his head and responded that he seemed to remember something, but seemed to be implying that he did not know." A "hit" head, and "She Moved Through the Fair",[1] as would the jack with the wood of the match bowled by my father on a Belfast park bowling green as if at "Belmont Gardens"[2] - "well on the Technical side" indeed: the 'butterfly' thus "Moved" to a "much better" place; 'the day' was his with "a friend in Bedford", my choice of destination for the "sixty-sixth": "Old Warden"; "God rest you" "Marchington (behind Wellington)": Irish "INTERNATIONAL" Tom Kennedy.

"Bowler runs off with another bowler's wife"? "La Belle Alliance" /"A damn close run thing" – "a little circumstance of village scandal" for Kennedy, as Edward Hilton might have concluded?

Authorities unworthy of the title simply promote themselves; those worthy promote awareness: "an English worthy", concluded Churchill; "and though advised of the position", lied the "sure" dictator: "Herewith [the day after the contracts were signed: "As speed is of the essence of the matter"] is the will and ["because of the difficulties of the family Home Protection

[1]   60th Feis Ceoil baritone first prize (She Moved Through the Fair /Blow, Blow Thou Winter Wind)

[2]   "God rest you merry – let nothing you dismay! As ever…"

Act"] …we want to be sure that this …was not a family home" –
"the difficulty which arises is that ...for about the last five years
Mr. Ewing has been spending most of his time at Abbeyville"
/"From time to time one or other of the children of the marriage
did spend time in the house with Ewing and one of them spent
a fairly long time there…" Subsequently: "he contemplated as
a very distinct possibility or probability that K…y would end
up by owning part or all of his lands. He would not be deterred
by that probability." Indeed: "part or all" thus as "possibility
or probability"; rather than "part" "possibility", indeed: "all"
"probability" – academic probability theory being "the essence
of the matter", versus kind consideration.

Nobody's business

"There must be specific procedure by
which to validate finality orders."
Petition excerpt, February 2019

"Shall I tell them now?" History can: the more truculent and grasping Hitler became in 1938, the more Chamberlain could influence the German people.

"I [AJP Taylor] have never been troubled by the dogmas of others about what history should be or how it should be written.

Most of this is sales talk by academics anxious to justify their existence. My view is that they should get on with writing books in their way and I will get on with writing them in mine. I have always been conscious of the artificiality of history. We sort human beings into national or class categories, when in reality each one of them is unique." "He [Chamberlain] was frankly contemptuous of the wishful thinking about the League in which it was fashionable in some quarters to indulge, and made no effort to conceal his feeling."

"But there is a reason that stream of consciousness is rarely used in works of political science..."[1] – "exceptional indeed and there is..." The 'rat', "being technical": "the sub-division application would of course put them on notice but there is a separate agreement for the sale back of the house and five acres."

---

[1]   Kirkus media book review

"He [judge C...y] earnestly urged Mr. Ewing to appoint a
legal team, so that the facts could be presented in legal fashion,
and ...said to ...e: [senior counsel] 'Get this sorted out ...out
of court'!!" He could not refer to the non-payment of £45,000
(one of the seven technical problems of the sale, none of which
were related by lawyers to Mr Ewing), for that issue was
pleaded by Mr Ewing, thus he referred to the non-application
to the Land commission (as introductory to advising Mr Ewing
to appoint 'legal advice'). Indeed, "it was fashionable in some
quarters to indulge" "in Latin" and to "sort human beings into
...categories": the educated class always has much to say, only
as blame-game professionals they never mean what they say, as
Mr Ewing ultimately noted concerning delays: "Was judge C...y
responsible?" The £45,000 issue thus cornered the 'rats', such
as reported to St Brendan's church concerning the negligence
panel solicitor's truculence against the £45,000 issue: "Indeed,
was this not the problem? That Robert Ewing was too much on
the ball and knew too much..." And indeed, "that stream of
consciousness" approach, untroubled "by the dogmas of others"
such as simply confuse: "The more Hitler was 'appeased' the
more truculent and grasping he became. It was quite clear that
war could not be long delayed..." Political science work is best
forwarded by 'a man of letters', and not indeed by "Alphabetical's
coming home."

"Dear [housing minister's private] Secretary,

I appreciate your time on this, however I should clarify
that I am concerned with performance of public policy, and
while the government may be continually under siege in the
Dail concerning ministerial performance, the situation on the
ground is the real area where we are quite routinely failed –

you can ensure such things as local elections and consultation rooms at council offices, but the public must also have a means to communicate directly, because such areas as county council are only media news when there are many bad roads – money fixes such problems, usually in advance, but there is generally no impetus for council to consider individual cases, or for local TDs to do anything but ask the council for a report, and which effectively is convenient to pass to the complainant – a routine that exists between legal professionals also, so the citizen is generally without a voice except when convenient to State component. The housing policy should be that roads serve homes first and foremost, as not even a secretary lives in his or her minister's pocket, and presidents of the State are only in residence for four years – the housing policy includes inhabited protected structures, and there is really nothing I can say to the council and its heritage section that will generate interest in high policy. I would advise that attention is given to the complaint process; council notes are not procedural as a complaint mechanism, and as with the legal profession, where there is no specific procedure to process complaint against system component, the components themselves tend to reply as if it is not in the interests of the State and the common good to acknowledge individual cases – the whole complaints procedure for components is also compromised because judgments by courts have no validation process – thus the top of the complaint process has no cap, so-to-speak, as if we are an oil company that does not truly want supply. I would ask you to send my kind consideration for the minister, and advice such as Walter Bagehot published for ministers in 1872 – I am of the opinion that the Irish State has spent precious little time examining such studies; and the government would do well to find some component that respects the dwelling concerned here – the Dail is not home to anyone, and some buildings are landmark and are home; politically, the government must perform housing and all the considerations involved, but there are outstanding issues that even the homeless regard as essential tasks, and I would advise that while government is not about good deeds relative to individual cases, there is one important good deed, and that is to acknowledge the individual case.

PS Bagehot basically refers to using one's common sense, which in his society was once related concerning the common law as "the common sense of the community, crystallised and formulated by our forefathers"; the legal business is against common sense and therefore against the common law, for there is business in negating law, just as there is little prestige in engineering if the ordinary citizen can identify the issues – one need only employ one's common sense to the road issue, but for that reason we may have no component interest – common sense is the unwelcome customer, and Bagehot was thus proved correct; we have "The people's garden", but that is no reason to hand the rest of the country over to 'victorian' bureaucracies."

Acknowledged by the justice minister's private secretary, July 2019, concerning the exploitative advice and judgment culture:

"Government is a manifestation of leadership and necessarily does not routinely declare its decisions by way of also relating the considered facts. In other words, the State executive is entitled to believe and behave as if knowing best.

Legal affairs are also government, and the legal profession would like to be entitled to believe and behave as if knowing best.

In other words, lawyers neither necessarily seek nor routinely relate the facts, and judges do not routinely base their decisions on the facts: the profession attempts to govern the client or litigant, rather than allow true executive status to the public.

Performing public responsibility generates a State system culture of seeking accurate information. Therefore, above all State components, the executive works by way of seeking accurate information. In other words, while State executive decision can be routinely trusted, the advice or decision of legal professionals cannot: the public, as the least responsible for public affairs and, therefore, the least orientated toward accurate information, is exploited: "as almost half the holding is going in the present proposed transfer".

The client knew "almost half" was somewhat of an exaggeration yet did not question the advice; indeed the public has no cultural routine to receive accurate information, or to even consider that accurate information is the routine sought context for executive decisions. In other words, the public tends to rely on component information, and its belief in the legal profession is exploited. The public needs to consider how the State executive works; and the State executive needs to more closely monitor the legal profession:

Robert Ewing wrote to Taoiseach Haughey as a consequence of solicitor non-availability learnt previous to dispute. He wrote while a co-defendant to civil litigation caused by that non-availability, and concerning the dispute caused by that non-availability. Subsequently, two court orders state appearance only for his co-defendant, William Ewing, because of that non-availability.

The letter reported negligence panel solicitor: "They are not taking any notice" of Mr Ewing who sought the negligence action (concerning solicitor who, as discovery would show, did not take any notice of him as client: "the theft" of Mr Ewing's lands), and the solicitor subsequently wrote to him contradicting earlier letter to him, inadvertently thus proving the report correct.

Subsequent to the litigation and Mr Ewing's passing, the Supreme court replied subsequent to its judgment that the negligence panel solicitor had not been provided with opportunity to act for Mr Ewing. Statement of claim mentioned that reply as provided with "absolutely no explanation whatsoever"; the only explanative aspect was that the judgment reads: "but subsequently the Ewings served a further notice of change of solicitors as a result of which..."

The said "further" solicitors - engaged subsequent to the negligence solicitor, withdrew after hearing; indisputably, therefore, opportunity was provided to defend Mr Ewing, contrary to what the first Supreme court would state, not only concerning the statement of no appearance, but most specifically thus:

> "In each case, it is clear that the supposed intentions of these defendants [the negligence panel solicitor and the previous solicitor] are claimed to have been frustrated by the action of their dismissal. As against the sixth defendant, [the subsequent solicitor] an identical allegation is made..."

Indeed, not only was the "sixth defendant" responsible for the orders which state appearance only for Mr Ewing, but they withdrew. Mr Haughey's minister for justice, and neither

Supreme court, stated anything both accurate and significantly relevant: unjustly, "the Ewings" to pay for the non-availability. Documents..."

Attempt to counter solicitor colleague deference – convenience to one-another's business, could not succeed when judges defer to lawyers rather than process, just as politicians and administrators defer to component reports, as if the component term for citizen is "loose cannon": "You only have to say somebody's unbalanced or mentally unstable..."

Mr Ewing noticed the nasty manner by which the "rat" replied deceitfully to judge Cassidy: "*Yes he did!*" "Mr Robert Ewing may be mistaken as to the manner" – the legal profession does not remark on its manner; therefore submission that manner is clearly that of "the nasty boys" – of the "dreadful [not justifiable] thing to say", is not accepted; reply would be termed: "shows how misunderstandings may arise" /"legal submissions employing these terms [procedural for 'striking out' pleadings] may tend to sound hurtful, aggressive or insensitive in the mouths of lawyers in a way which is not necessarily intended." It was nobody's business that lawyer submissions can be deceitful.

And what 'is not necessarily intended' by media? "Of course, Prince Charles is not a member. More probably he is mouthing something..." More probably a member: "Charles Windsor" in New York, "calling from a pay-phone down the street." Minister: "I bet you wrote that Holden!" Such is probability culture 'in the driving-seat': "I was very cynical about Diana." /"Is there some [parliamentary] anxiety that she's something of 'a loose cannon'?" No cultural possibility of identifying "the nasty boys" as 'loose cannon', rather the latter term applied relative to natural relation such as statehood is not evolved to:

"Her reaction was really one of astonishment, I mean: *why is this being said – why are people wanting to do this – what do I have to do?"* /"A public department is very apt to be dead to what is wanting for a great occasion till the occasion is past." Such is media and component report culture generally, product not of times present but times past: "It [the wedding] was to be held in St Paul's cathedral and not the more traditional Westminster Abbey." /"More than 30 years ago…"

About it

"Choice, not chance, decides destiny."
Parliamentary private secretary *Rawat*[1]

Tánaiste Frances Fitzgerald had a popular reputation but lied to the Dáil and resigned: as minister for justice she had tolerated garda 'dirty-tricks' against a garda whistle-blower. I wrote to her while she was minister for justice; yet I kept the letter, and opened it after she resigned, to see why:

"To Frances Fitzgerald,

Garda as State snoop on the citizen only get bored and involved in local victimization with the exploitative citizen bent on grabbing and averting their own boredom.

Remove Garda from citizen policing – teach *personal responsibility* to the citizen, rather than generate the problems by the pretence that the State 'looks after us all'.

Police target areas: traffic/road safety etc. No more targeting of citizens as sought by the exploitative element – 'the devil take the hindmost' routine as pursued by solicitors in the belief that the State will always back them up – 'police State' over the citizen's moral-backbone.

Robert Ewing

---

[1] PPS Rawat (December 10th 1957-)

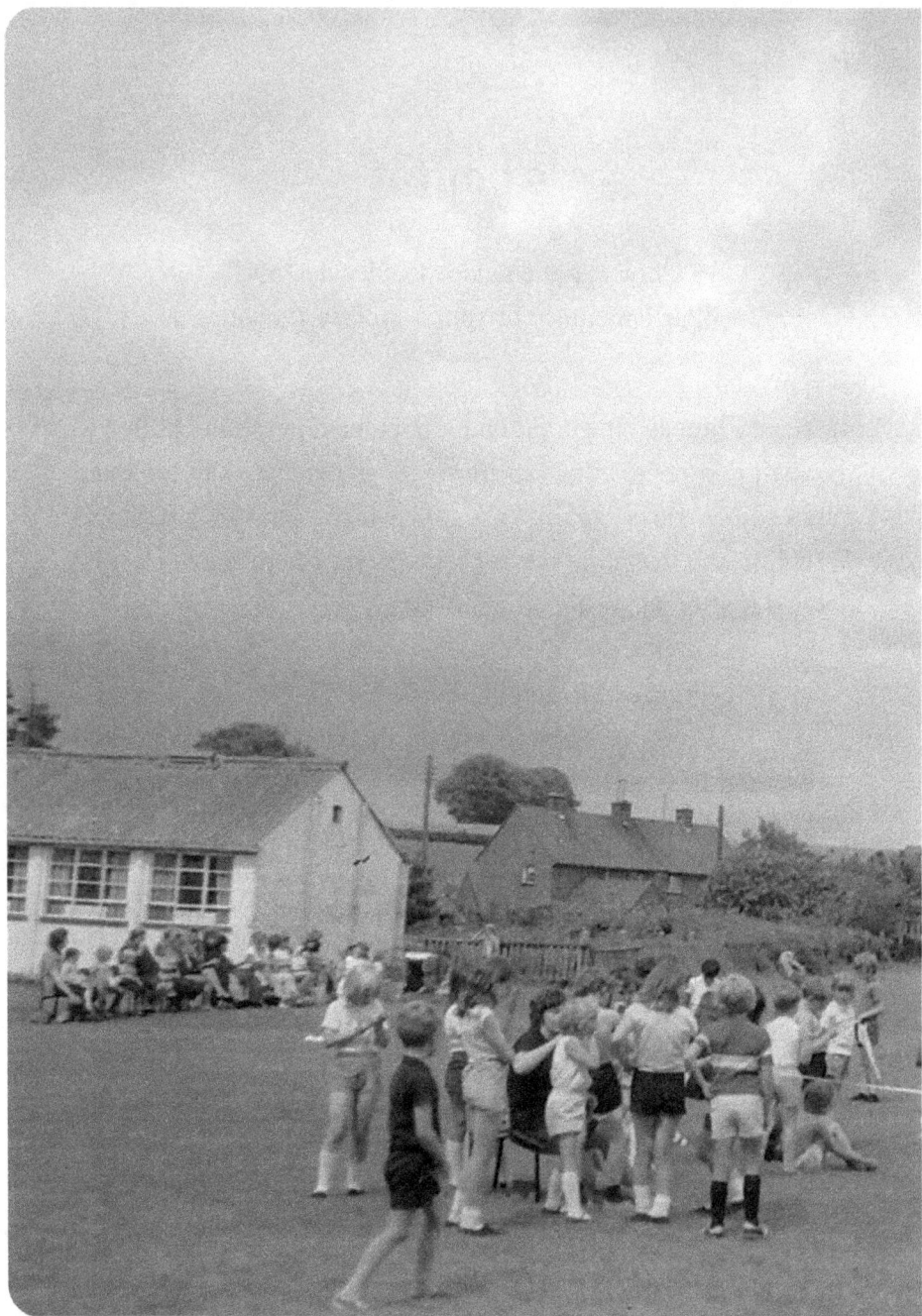

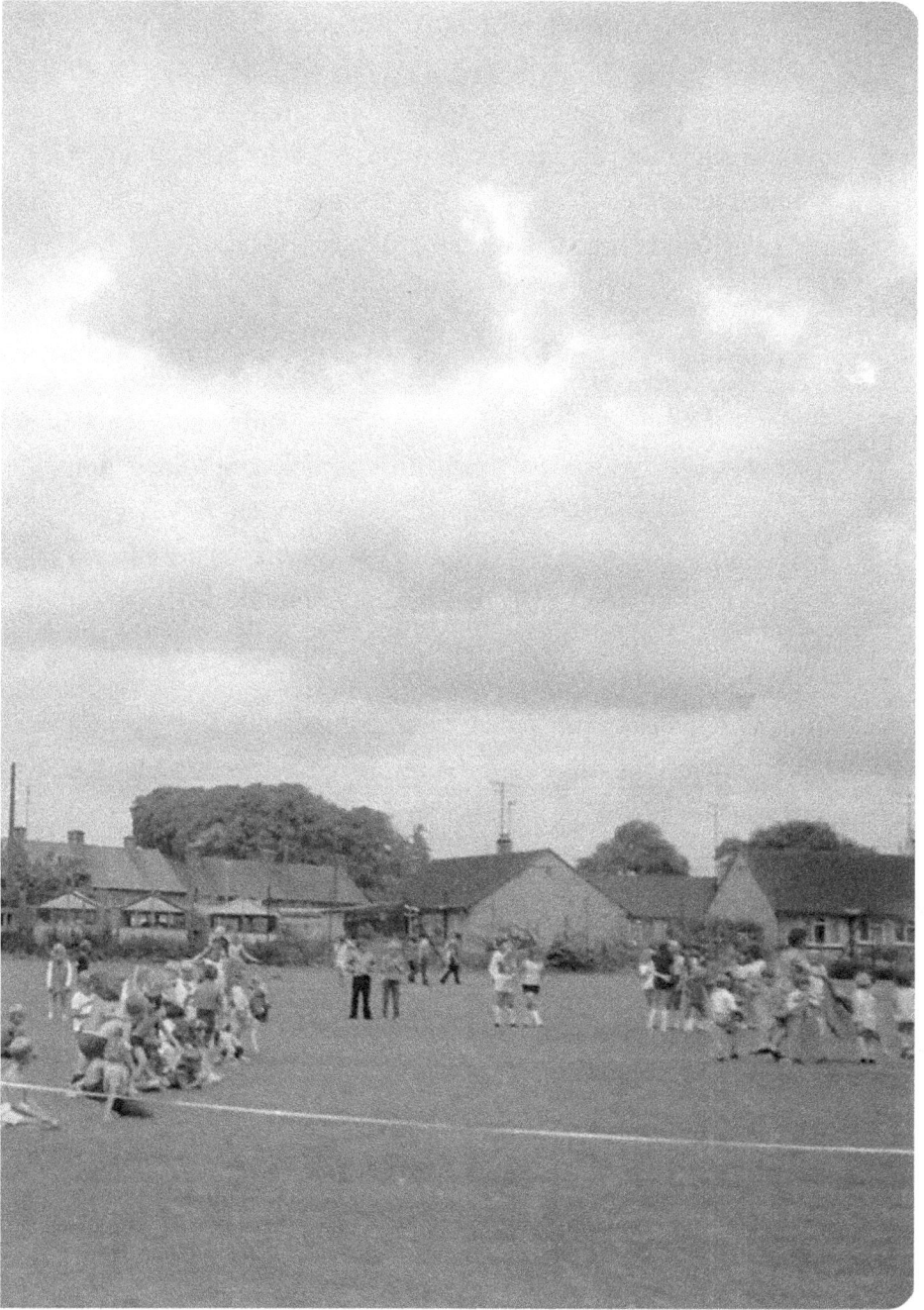

P.S. *Politically difficult*: Garda wanted in their present position of 'nanny State', providing the middleclass with their voice 'on the street'. *Garda*: middleclass 'pet', money to rule over community, as is inclination of solicitors.

Garda boredom – useful to the middleclass

> - entertainment generated from putting the citizen 'in the dock' without 'a solicitor'. Middleclass interest that Garda are bored. Solicitor participation: invention of client relation /defendant relation etc. See the entertainment problem as 'Rome Rule' on a wet day."

Neither referees nor police are whistle-blowers as an entertainment, but it is too late now, of course, to advise that politician (as might perpetuate "a popular reputation"), that "Mussolini got bored."[1]

"Late, late show", this is, but "what a show!" "In war, whichever side may call itself the victor, there are no winners but all are losers."

Courage: "But in a miscellaneous world, there is now one evil…"
"R-of-way to be protected in any event."
State lie: "Robert Ewing now says…"
"Austen's peace".

---

[1]   USA service information film 3

"We, the German Führer and Chancellor and the British Prime Minister, have had a further meeting today and are agreed in recognising that the question of Anglo-German relations is of the first importance for the two countries and for Europe."

"You've never been to Aspen, I suppose";[1] "to represent effectually general sense in opposition to bureaucratic sense";[2] "his species must be his own".

Poets: "the unacknowledged legislators", because they "forge social sympathies"[3] – challenge the divisiveness of politics?

Merlin (major-general to the second cavalry brigade of the first cavalry corps) was said to be *Swiftsure* ("the suggestion ...that I overbore ...is utterly without foundation, is absolute nonsense and has been made up"); only on the other side, "with Mr. Neville Chamberlain at Waterloo",[4] was a Griffin (an infantryman's immediate reply to Napoleon's 'one trick pony'): "Here come these fools again."

Consistency: "But in a miscellaneous world, there is now one evil, and now another."

"The right-of-way ...was mine since 1973 ...I told her that I had purchased the right ...with the lands and that my Solicitor would clarify this ...if she needed clarification."

State lie: "Robert Ewing now says..." /"He now says..."

No. 2 Butterfly stamp.

---

[1] Richard Nixon
[2] Walter Bagehot (1872)
[3] Shelley's opinions
[4] Keith Gordon

"We regard the Agreement signed last night and the Anglo-German Naval Agreement as symbolic of the desire of our two peoples never to go to war with one another again."

Poetry: "One cannot legislate for more", "and we're much better"?

Misunderstanding is generally known to travel fastest, with but one exception: our default (or 'fáilte'). "Surely civil, constitutional and criminal law must be conducted on separate 'Inis' days in this country – a culture of diary and interest..."

Of interest to dying Neville Chamberlain at the Duke of Wellington estate (his opinion being: "never for one moment have I had any doubt that I had to do what I did"): "I call it improper pride to let fools' notions hinder you from doing a good action."[1] "The action is brought for an improper purpose, and not for the assertion of legitimate rights", lied the 'one trick pony' - "expressly".

And logic: "But in a miscellaneous world, there is now one evil and now another. The very means which best helped you yesterday, may very likely be those which most impede you to-morrow – you may want to do a different thing to-morrow, and all your accumulation of means for yesterday's work is but an obstacle to the new work."[2]

"Present position is as if I am retransferring to Bill without getting anything for it."

State lie: "Robert Ewing now says..." /"He now says..." /"Here, such quotation is necessary simply to set out his case as pleaded. The references to the "defendant" ["Here, he sued only

---

[1]   Middlemarch by "George Eliot" - Mary Ann Cross
[2]   Walter Bagehot (1872)

Ireland and the Attorney General as defendants"] ...are both to Ireland and the Attorney General."

The Custom House library.

"We are resolved that the method of consultation shall be the method adopted to deal with any other questions that may concern our two countries, and we are determined to continue our efforts to remove possible sources of difference and thus to contribute to assure the peace of Europe."

Wellington retreating to Waterloo commented: "I suppose in England they will say we have been licked." Only he could not have legislated for more than John Colborne's legitimate rights, such as my action was fought for (class ruler at hand for measuring, not for striking hands[1]): not improper purpose at hand, and blame-game at hand, and "misunderstandings" at hand, rather evolution at hand, and the individual case at hand, and the outstanding quality at hand: "fáilte"; the choice, not chance, that is at hand: the Griffon:

> "I graduated ["in Coventry in 1962 as a Student Apprentice studying Mechanical Engineering"] and moved in 1967 to Perkins Engines in Peterborough as an Applications Engineer in their Technical Office. A small office with about 5 engineers ...After 5 years in this office I moved to Field Test at Perkins and in 1978 moved to JCB Excavators in Uttoxeter. I was specialising in NVH (noise, vibration & harshness) and in 1982 moved to a specialist acoustic company."

---

[1] Striking the future ordained Francis for helping less intelligent pupils

"I recall your father with great affection, a truly lovely man who adored his family. I was sorry that we never met up again" – "how much I enjoyed working with him." /"We worked in the same office for about 5 years between 1968 and 1973 but … weren't exactly colleagues working closely together …he was just a very good friend. Someone …I loved. A real gentleman."

"A small office with about 5 Engineers doing calculations on engine performance, and of course Bill Ewing, who kept us all sane with his dry humour, ready wit and the ability to avoid doing anything in a rush and[1] …if at all. We watched the effect this had on our frenetic boss [the Merlin] with great satisfaction and delighted in hearing his ["Bill's"] wonderful ["wonderful, descriptive"] excuses!"

The battle between "possible sources of difference", on the one hand, and on the other hand: "most conscientious and attentive to his duties"; "fools" and "fools' notions" on the one hand, and on the other hand: "it is with extreme regret that we have had to release him from our service"; "always making bricks without straw",[2] on the one hand, and on the other hand: "always had excellent control of staff"; "a permanent battle ground", on the one hand, and on the other hand, "leave free the energies of mankind" - "the new work"; the "damage he has caused" to Isis.

---

[1] Reply to Ian Jones: "Dad played some piano at junior school but refused to play the march for the class to march into the school; I entirely agree with your use of the word "sane", and tend to think that his refusal to play the march was an early example of it." Reply to Robert Ewing: "While you are working your life is fairly regimented…"

[2] Salisbury (1886)

"I[1] have looked at Abbeyville House on the Buildings of Ireland website and it is fascinating as Dad ["dear old Bill" – "your father …had wisdom, and modesty and humour. *Wonderful qualities that I would so enjoy sharing with him now*"] was always talking about it."

"Dad was always talking about it"?

Well, butterfly, that *is* about it.

Means/Ends

---

[1]   "Powys" to the people – Ian Jones to Robert Ewing, February 2018

Acknowledgements

"It was so kind of you to take the trouble to write
as you did." *The Prince of Wales* to Robert Ewing[1]

My great thanks to Loughrea Printing Works for their help in assembling this book as first conveyed to Authorhouse.

Of the university element contributory to my writing and research, the person to single out for particular mention is he who at junior school had his glass of paintbrush water twice accidently knocked over his painting by an elbow of mine as I passed by ("I was just passing" /"I was just going past").[2]

Our headmaster was presiding, and was simply 'bad news' concerning the first "Passing By", and therefore I anticipated 'worse news' and decided for a "Silent Worship"[3] exit to my home, such was my immediate view that misunderstanding must generally travel fastest and that he had not yet knocked about that subject. He was no Dr. Peden: "The responsibility for errors is, of course, the author's."

"Gouverner, c'est choisir." Ultimately, my university friend was confident that I would join the discussion subject: Bristol Rearmament and the Treasury, 1932-1939; so thank you Dorothy Bastick; and thank you Ian (or Iain) Jones.

---

[1] September 12th 2016
[2] Writers Jay and Lynn
[3] Father's record

I also particularly thank the "UL" at Cambridge and "Joe" University, Birmingham, for their kind co-operation, without which the much knocked about subject of 'appeasement' might have had to join the queue of "PREM" academics at the "PRO" (London).

My published work called "Abbeyville House" began with reference to local "'pastures green' and 'quiet waters by'" enhanced by relative quiet and a neglected cut-stone field-bridge. Authorhouse effectively related the commonality of these projects by stating of this work: "Written in a stream-of-consciousness style[1] ...it will cause readers to pause and think deeply."

---

[1] "You have written an innovative book with a distinctive style. Its subject matter is both informative and provocative." /"Written in a stream-of-consciousness style and based on many observations from your life, it will cause readers to pause and think deeply."

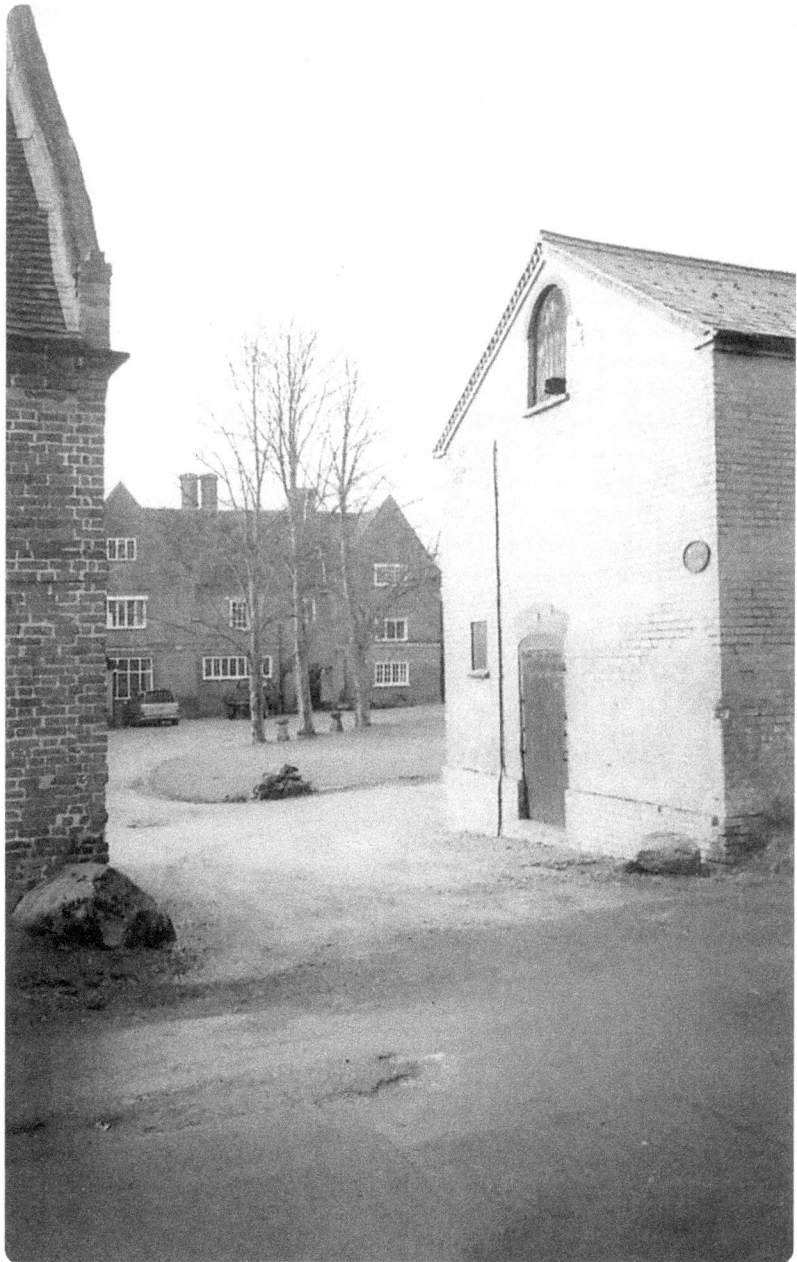

Appendix

**Notes of 4th June 2004 /22nd August 2006
/8th March 2007 /8th December 2014**

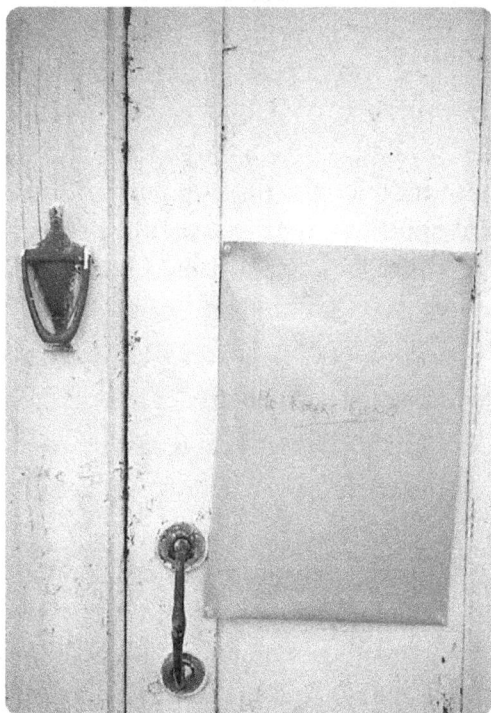

**"It is my experience that Eire …paper rights
are what Irish business wipes its backside on."**

/4-6th January 2020 /9th April 2020

EDUCATING CEAUSESCU
Originally a note headed by its date

Is there a country where great public buildings are never seen? Where the poorer of its citizens are consulted when the idea of a great public building is being entertained? Where the great do not proclaim their greatness through an exploitation of the people, but rely instead on the dynamic of their own ideas? Such a country would become a progressive society, focused on the wellbeing of individuals. Institutions that live primarily for themselves and oppose change in an effort to survive would not exist. Such a country's greatness would be found in its people, rather than in its public buildings.

When a country's poorer citizens have the power to veto the building of structures which do not reflect their standard of living and fail to enhance their stature within society, then, and only then, will the cycle of revolution end because power will have come to truly lie with the people.

Perhaps our great artistic structures should be admired. But on whose shoulders were they built? And who decides on the burden? They stand as monuments to inequality, and to the shortened lives of many. And they function today as they have always functioned, to draw power away from the individual and give it to a small ruling minority. Making the hardest work pay the least and honesty pay even less.

Power thrown away brings corruption. The friend of the professional crook is an artistic extravagance beside the public road. As people we walk in. But as peasants we walk out. Robbed of our individual worth, and always out of pocket. Corruption awaits at every turn. Material greatness achieves its own reward.

THE SPIN OF BALLY-GO-BACKWARDS
Originally a note to Letters at the Galway Advertiser

Did you hear about the Kerry-man suicide bomber who intended to blow up a plane in mid-air? When his bomb failed to detonate he jumped out without a parachute.

People write to you from time to time in order to expose some failing on the part of a community or nation, yet it is individuals that do wrongful acts, and pointing the finger forever away from individual responsibility toward some greater cultural or ethnic failing has never succeeded to uproot wrongdoing either at home or abroad. To attempt to actually uproot wrongdoing would be to unsettle more than just the focus of our resentments, for it would lead to an unwelcome analysis of our own failings, and it is that neglect to examine failures at home that ultimately keeps the trouble going abroad – since every nation claims guardianship of international peace.

My proposal for world peace has therefore nothing to do with lecturing others, but instead centres on leading by example – meaning that every individual must have direct procedural access to make their views known on matters that affect them at local government level (therefore offering an immediate alternative to making the issue either a political or a legal one). If such facility existed it would not only remove countless misunderstandings between individuals and their authorities, it would in some cases provide an outlet for the bruised emotions of likely suicide cases, and would, indeed, help bring down the suicide rate –

and thus ultimately would help bring down the suicide bomber. It is individuals, indeed, who lead communities astray, and the global war that has existed for countless centuries will not cease, indeed, until peace loving citizens stop pussy footing around Eden lecturing perennial weeds with the buzz of their lawnmowers, but put their hoes to work against such like instead – as a honourable politician once said: "The plough is mightier than the pen, just as the pen is mightier than the sword." It is the plough then to which we must turn if we wish to turn over a new leaf for this world, rather than to those who are apt to fail to call a spade a spade and have so far, indeed, forgotten what the good old garden hoe was designed for – in their preference, indeed, for an application of condescending words that merely serves to poison international relations still further.

Indeed, we all believe we know what the problems are abroad, but when it comes to recognising the contribution of our own society to them we look toward our flowerbeds for some welcome distraction, forgetting that charity begins at home, and abroad is really no different than Kerry. How many disputes between individuals stem from that exact failing to identify imperfections on both sides of their boundary wall?

The Kerry-man I talked to on the subject of procedural obstructions against complaints agreed the present state of evasion and obstruction against victims of insensitive local government departments to be an evil. Let us therefore have adequate procedures of complaint. Then perhaps one day complaints both at home and abroad will have their answer short of bombs and bullets – the villain for which remains the pointed non-green finger that is but the spin of Bally-go-backwards poisoning us all.

HUMAN RIGHTS
– THE LACK OF PUBLIC CONCERN
Originally a note to Amnesty International

It is my experience that Eire does not offer a completely comprehensive legal service and does not wish to address that fact. The reason for this gap in the legal system is firstly, that solicitors never need to explain why they turn down certain clients, and secondly there are a great number of solicitors willing to pretend that they are happy to take on certain clients when in reality they simply endeavour to manipulate a case in accordance with what suits them from a business point of view – something they can do with great confidence because the system denies client access to barristers without solicitor introduction, and the judiciary does its best to treat solicitors and barristers as being beyond reproach, as if the academic law world applies to the real law world – something that simply is not true, because business interests imposes limitations on how much law is pleaded in the courts.

What all this means is that in certain cases there is opposition within the legal profession itself against the law being brought forward in them. In my family's case the doings of a former solicitor were not examined in accordance with the facts, in a legal case that his former firm had an obvious business interest in, and the opposition within the legal profession against such facts was clearly in part linked to the fact that the former solicitor had been made a judge of the District Court. He appeared a witness in the case, and the case greatly affected my family's home.[1]

I provide this note to Amnesty International today because I believe there is a human rights issue involved here, and I believe the general public must some day come to realise that the firm basis of human rights is the law, and without a comprehensive legal service no-one's human rights are safeguarded. My endeavour is therefore not simply to have my own human rights secured, but see that the general public appreciates that the present legal system is a denial, to certain victims of abuse, of their means to address their abuse. The hope for my family at present is that there is a human rights lawyer who will recognise the human rights issue NOW and not leave it to the present system to make its own impression on that fact – the present system being rooted firmly against there being a recognition that some human rights issues arise through the abuse of the legal system from within the legal profession (in our case such abuse began with the former solicitor, continued through ten years of litigation and three additional legal firms, and today is in its twentieth year – applications to the European Court of Human Rights having so far been made in appalling conditions and without, I think, a proper awareness within Europe that national tribunals now have every reason to overlook such human rights issues, because THEIR VIEWS are required by the Court, and in our case – to take an example, our concern for our home was presented by the State as a concern for land, and obviously land is not a human rights issue!

---

[1] Supreme Court lies, subsequently: "Robert Ewing's view is that ["the pressures of"] …the litigation badly affected his father's health." Contract law quoted by William Ewing: "the person adversely affected"

HUMAN RIGHTS COMMISSION
Originally a note to the Éire State HRC

I am Plaintiff concerning this residence, in negligence proceedings against the State. I write to you on that subject and on related subjects concerning human rights, in order that you may be able to assist me.

The underlying grievance is that the legal profession obstructs our right to challenge claims concerning this dwelling. The principal claim is for access through the domestic yard that until domestic alterations by me would involve coming between the backdoor of the house and the toilet.

The European Court of Human Rights correspondence to me involved misunderstanding and a request for clarification, and there was obviously an assumption that the access sought did not have domestic consequences. I was disappointed that human rights machinery made assumption of that nature, but of course not every application to the machinery is grounded on basic comprehension of the Convention.

I believe however that the said correspondence might well represent a confirmation that judges of the court tend to be influenced by the national judges; in other words, if the national judges, as occurs in the matter of the dwelling, say that the case concerns land, it is more likely that the application will be rejected. This is an important point because it must be considered that State laws are not convenient to everyone, and attempts are made by legal professionals every day to evade some part of the law; if the legal controversy might possibly invite judgment against the State in connection to legal professional conduct at any level, the controversy is better minimised, such as by not properly advising the victim, and such as by representing to the State that the conflict is about land. In these terms, the existence of human rights can be an onerous liability on the very people they are supposed to protect.

The theory of human rights involves that individuals are provided with the essentials to enable them to earn their living; for example, the individual unable to sleep at night for aircraft noise is unemployable during the day. I have had no reasonable opportunity to earn a living since I moved here in 1984, and the dwelling is in a ruinous condition relative to the problems; the situation has continually worsened with every remedy applied, as the claims on the dwelling derive from control connected to solicitor fraud. I reported the "theft" of the property and the inclination of independent solicitors to perpetuate it, to Taoiseach [Charles] Haughey, and Discovery order resulted in us [the succession] obtaining the proof of the theft.

It might be argued that while solicitors tend to generate business for one-another by generating cases, that sooner or later they would inadvertently generate the involvement of the Court of Human Rights, but the key consideration involved is that convenience tends to dictate, and the national judges tend to be guided by their professional colleagues – there would be no acknowledgement of inconvenient case, and therefore no colleague pleads one. The Convention concerns both the most serious and relatively trivial issues on assumption of national legal advice and professionalism, but since that assumption is wrong, the Convention is wrong. Those transported in cattle-trucks and gassed or shot [reference to the holocaust] were thinking only of their right to life; their call for human rights did not involve protection from aircraft noise or right to privacy; no-one supposes that Member States of the European Union need law to prevent them from torturing individuals; what then lies between those extremes of uninvited wedding photographs and torture? What averts the likely serious threat to individuals within the context of the origin being business fraud? In those terms the Convention is indeed wrong, just as the [Éire] State was wrong to create the Land Commission – even while being avoided (transfer of entirety of lands primarily from [harasser] fear of Land Commission acquisition of the fields sought), and even while subjected to further irregularities (consent sought without agreement of the vendor to sub-divide the lands as agreed at the time of the contract and transfer), the Commission provided what the irregular application sought, as if the concept that a number of people might find the Commission inconvenient, and might find a solicitor to advise them accordingly, had never crossed the State's mind. This dwelling was transferred in such a sale and remains transferred thirty-four years later because [Éire] paper rights are what Irish [Éire] business wipes its backside on.

DISTINCTION versus EXTINCTION
Originally a note to interviewer Rick Bell

"Hello, and welcome to a Top Gear [Clarkson, May and Hammond – "we're here because we're going to have a race" – a human race – "we've got a choice"] special!" In other words: "Some things are meant to be…"

One aspect of this book is to alert the non-colonizing educated class individual against risking anyone mistaking the honest deployment of class terminology as the dishonest deployment. This was particularly indicated by way of quoting Al Gore and regional Irish Supreme Court.

Hammond: "And if Al Gore is to be believed…" /"And then to make matters worse", review of this book is like a white-wash: "even an extended passage on a property dispute…" The author clearly relates 'testing' of both State and media. Does the nature of the review relate effectively that a media exclusion of comment subsequently described by the internet machinery: "Detected as spam", constitutes white-wash? In other words: both media responses detectable as white-wash, and the review effectively "even an extended passage" of the exclusion? Effectively extending a colleague's opinion is legal professional culture. The review does not state of the origin of this book: 'the evidence from historical research and legal controversies', rather: "this book, which has its origin in the comments" to the website of a "Irish magazine that covers current affairs and culture"; the principal aspects of the evidence could not be directly related to the public via posting to the website, and unlikely received otherwise except via independent publication, contrary to the said claim: "covers"; the evidence validates principal comments; and since the review supposedly validates the reviewer's opinion by way of quotation, the reviewer almost certainly could discern the same origin of quotation by the author, yet the review reads 'deaf, dumb and blind' to his evidence and, therefore, is "spam" - as said of the exclusion.

"But there is a reason that stream of consciousness is rarely used in works of political science:"? Hammond: "Well, hang on, [the author did not argue about political science] so …we'd [the wed of "Some things are meant to be"] …stand in line … it's a silly test, I'm not doing that." "But" State and media are sufficiently interested to respond appropriately to the public? No need for citizens to allege to mankind generally concerning State or media?

Historian Somervell wrote: "He formed his own picture of the situation, and it turned out to be fundamentally mistaken", as explanation for premier Chamberlain opting to direct foreign policy: "He became on major issues the director"; however, only as required by "the situation", which "turned out" almost as dangerous as feared (American public opinion was slow to discern the common danger). Somervell, like the book reviewer, "formed his own picture of the situation, and it turned out to be fundamentally mistaken." The author understood that the public will not read a hundred pages of evidence no-matter how advisable and edited.

Clarkson: "Tomorrow we hit the bolder field, [Hammond: "On the way he would encounter …cathedrals"] O.K.?" May: "What would those salmon eggs go really well with?" Clarkson replied: "Well, a crisp white..." Predators obtain salmon eggs, and digest them with 'a crisp white-wash'. The reviewer quoted what the author related to be "text messages", only the review thus implies that the so-called "legal case" was won (in other words: legal process obtained for "a property dispute"): "Huge respect 4 u guys..." The author related a continuing and fundamental procedural crisis relative to the law of Southern Ireland which, because many countries have the same system, has "INTERNATIONAL" significance, as also has the news of the post-war failure to honour Chamberlain, yet the review contradicts such significance as if the author merely relates a number of past controversies.

The government received report of a national crisis of also international significance from a regional State solicitor, who subsequently reported the response to the media, and justice minister Flynn's response was effectively a joke as related by the solicitor subsequent to the murder of a newspaper journalist in order to deny her evidence concerning the crisis being heard in court, therefore justice minister Owen, Flynn's successor, acknowledged the crisis. The government response then was to front-line the crisis, and Flynn was scapegoated for the State 'business as usual' which had invited the journalist to front-line the crisis. Justice minister Donoghue succeeded Owen and allowed the 'business as usual' against Robert Ewing's litigation concerning lawyer negation of legal process, most particularly at rehearing two weeks prior to the murder; both the account of the initial completed hearing and the evidence obtained by way of discovery order extending that hearing was negated by the rehearing, and the new order effectively relates this by stating counsel appearance for co-defendant William Ewing, and no appearance for his co-defendant, Robert Ewing, the discoverer that a solicitor was generating the property crisis. Justice minister Burke preceded Flynn and would not acknowledge the perpetuation of the crisis reported by Robert Ewing, to whom justice minister replied thirty years later with such 'business as usual' as Burke. Court registrar described lawyers generally as: "the jokers", and also commented: "The injustices that go on here!" Judges and justice ministers perpetuate lawyer jokes, effectively as commented by newspaper reporter to Robert Ewing: "It's all a con, isn't it?" And lawyer said that plaintiffs generally are not good characters. That opinion is from media, court service and legal profession such as the State and media refuse to relate officially; "a public duty to inform the public", 'joked' a newspaper lawyer explaining the demise of a court order inconvenient to the newspaper industry. Both State and media acknowledged the front-line attempted by solicitor Galvin and undertaken principally by journalist Guerin, but refuse to acknowledge the front-line undertaken by Robert Ewing, who as author therefore relates the said media disinclination to front-line a national crisis inconvenient to routine media reporting of news; he has that duty, just as he has the duty to refute the 'joke' that Mr Ewing's opponent was wronged.

News is not opinion, and therefore the news is not that "Ewing is a man with many opinions", rather he occupies the front-line against the media's attempt to control news and the legal profession's attempt to control legal opinion, neither of which challenges ministerial 'business as usual' except in the terms Somervell theorized: "party-political reasons" (as if "the situation" supposed by the mythology related the supposed failure "to offer the control of and responsibility for" British rearmament to Churchill). Somervell thus effectively related the origin of the present crisis: "the control" of news and legal opinion, and the "responsibility" of public duty indeed, undertaken by a number of specialists "who obviously knew more about such matters than anyone else", meaning, however, "such matters" generally, not necessarily "more" relevantly "than anyone else": "He [Churchill] was not asked." /"I [Edward Wood] have often wondered whether or how the course of history might have been changed if he [Chamberlain] had acted in the sense I suggested." Mankind has many opinions, and media attempt to obtain more of them was an origin of this book, only the reviewer lectured as if the author generated crisis: "It tends to make complicated subjects even more difficult to understand." The simplest subjects are the most difficult to understand, and misunderstanding generates crisis such as the reviewer experienced – the "challenging" consequences of complicated wandering of the wondering mind such as generated the opinion: "the course of history might have been" better, more likely: worse; a world of controversies and confusion such as Chamberlain visibly and indisputably challenged at Heston - 'Butterfly in the Well'. His "simplicity" was acknowledged, yet political science has rarely if ever supposed the validity of the simplest respectful explanation that he was a competent statesman; it must be noted that it is easier to complicate than simplify, and to lose than find one's way. And therefore the uninterested to understand will likely misunderstand; and that is the difference between the author and the mythology: "It was a logical policy logically pursued, though Chamberlain made some singularly foolish remarks in the course of his pursuit of it." The logic presumably being to pursue history, only he was employed for political science performance, not for a political science exam: "I [Hammond] shall be ...using traditional methods ...and here's why ...victory then would be mine."

Thus distinction versus extinction: the State and media should be required by law to offer citizens a voice, principally agreed 25-50 word summary of constituency consultation, and option too of publication in principal regional newspapers designated by ministerial appointment, thereby educating non-academic basics, effectively the 'street education' of male parent tuition which balances the female parent tuition of academic State basics which otherwise generate exploitable misconceptions concerning performance of public policy. If the survival of any human family or the ability to register what our ears and eyes receive involves generating balanced tuition between academic and non-academic State basics, both State and media should perform the balanced tuition. Allow suppression and oppression such as State and media 'business as usual' dictates, and society evolves to be 'deaf, dumb and blind', three little lost maids from school as a result of "spam", note "internet comment", "legal case", and "poem": "this internet comment relating to his father's legal case rewritten as a poem". Clarkson: "And to be honest our minds kept wandering..." Here are three found: "Evil triumphs when good men do nothing" /"Good man" (Roosevelt's telegram to Chamberlain concerning the Munich agreement, against which we hear: "Chamberlain did nothing") /"Nothing however happened," Chamberlain did nothing to offer creating "national government" until May 1940, "and I have often wondered whether or how the course of history might have been changed if he had", as if Munich ended the risk of negatively confused opinion - the principal threat to the strategic means by which to remedy the crisis; "good men" generally "do nothing" because they are too confused to know what to do, and not least because averting and remedying confusion is a most *simple* basic requirement of society only academic tuition "covers" this as "challenging", just as Wood failed to consider the simple concept that competent government triumphed throughout the dictator's rule, and just as academics failed to consider that Roosevelt combined simplicity with his "kindly expression of opinion": "Good man" – concept of Munich no different to what Hitler expressed, only he simply referred to the triumphant allies (who were 'three little maids' barred only from Southern Ireland, the region at one time named the Irish "Free State", and since that time Hitler's concept of a free State, its origin associated with a nationalist revolutionary war).

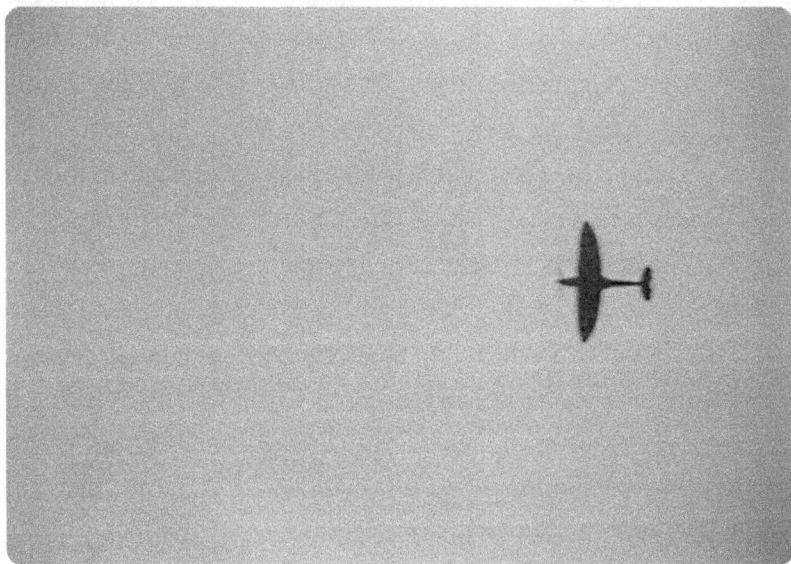

Mankind has many opinions, and media attempt to obtain more of them was an origin of this book, only the reviewer lectured as if the author generated crisis, and spam generates crisis.

Encouraging more opinions is not wrong, but encouraging more arguing is; mankind has many opinions, but rarely "Good man" is one of them, because the distinction of simplicity is generally subordinated to "kindly expression" meant to avert argument, only such subordination, while definable as 'a rule of spam', is increased by common profession, and such is not simply the inferior poetry but the threat of extinction, because mankind is thus not in the front-line, partisanship is: "You wouldn't be in this mess if you hadn't taken the law into your own hands"; the rule indeed of spam, even in reply to 'Good man' (June 1990), not just to the competent response to a crisis (May 1986); it may be very old news but it is not spam to relate that the voice of the human race is being subordinated to dictatorships, because that is "this mess" and it is a simple explanation continually subordinated indeed to 'business as usual'. We all have a choice, and it must be to resist the inclination of statehood to be the end rather than the means; the relevant publication process for distinction began in 1872; in other words, the author is a successor to Walter Bagehot.

FLANAGAN'S FIFTEEN MINUTES
Clue as to "the show ship" initialing "I.K.B."

Received by Authorhouse prior to the Covid-19 crisis: "chancing to envelop are engaged by choice" /"Humanity needs caring for, not exploitation our ...world" (23rd August 2019), and thereby related to the world during the crisis (24th March 2020): "HESTON, England [the publicity machine receives the 'butterfly', providing such "care" as Canning advised] – Myths, lies and confusion chancing to envelop our post-war world ..."

This is the only part of this book to acknowledge the health crisis, also the housing crisis said to have significantly influenced the electorate against voting for Mr Varadkar in 2020; "but it is too late now, of course, to advise that politician", "politically, the government must provide housing" – "home; politically," – "kind consideration for the minister, and advice" indeed against "hurtling through space on an unknown trajectory", but since the cultural 'business as usual' is indeed neither systemically nor culturally anybody's business to challenge, only you and I indeed "are home", against which the 'keeping the worst of things quiet' routines will always be too late - "2020 vision" was a chapter title concerning "Culture 2020" in the original concept of this book.

The concept of solicitor availability is partly that it reduces non-procedural confrontations – the "traditionary Irishman", yet the State is not concerned to ensure solicitor availability: the machinery is generally suited to keeping the worst of the component evil quiet. Guerin died partly relative to the same civility pretence within the State as she challenged from the underworld; both involve independence from the immediate consequences of such decisions as forwarded to me by a TD despite involving quote of my request to the writer to desist writing to me (predictably, the document stated nothing both accurate and significantly relevant). Gearán from John Searson: "seen and read the [pleaded] truth but [the judges] decided to lie." No "deeper interest" is "no direct interest" is no common interest is "that most astounding and troublesome of all" human phenomena, statehood: "our judiciary is renowned the world over" - justice minister Flanagan's "reassuring all" press release, "the art of categorization", 7th February 2020. Renown indeed: "it must now be understood" by the public that the media has yet to vindicate reliance on the media to challenge virus toxic public relations.

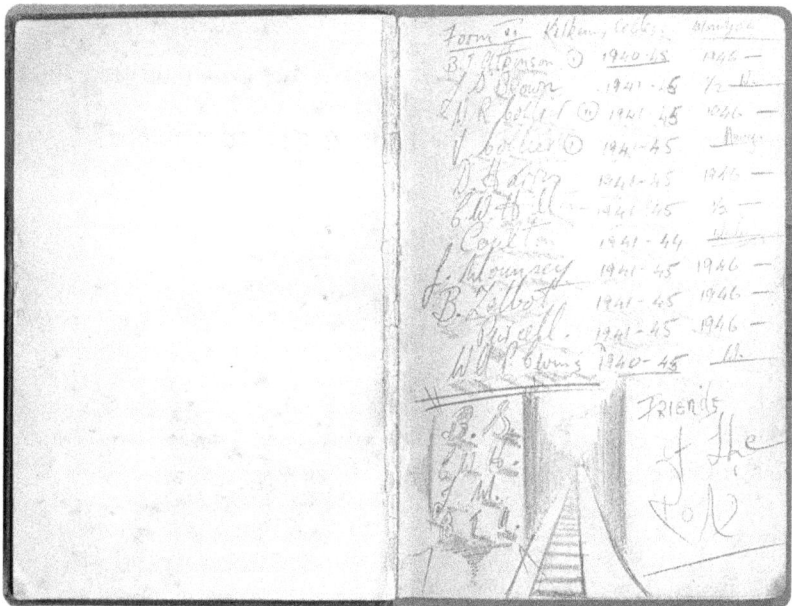

I
N
D
E
X

Village subject dates and commentators

February 29th 2016
The Crookedness of Irish Politics
Gunning for ideas   **Series of five, 73-74**
doofus 2016
ValerieMcDonald
MatCon
Robert Ewing

March 23rd 2016
Equality and Human Rights Commission
colour orange   **Series of four, 75**
two ronnies
natkingcola
Robert Ewing

April 20th 2016
1916 and the ongoing danger of conservative revolution
Revolving Staircase   **Series of seven, 77-78**
dog&bone   **and other: 149**
Just Mary   **149**
Robert Ewing
Joe Rooney to Revolving Staircase
Robert Ewing to Joe Rooney
Robert Ewing to Revolving Staircase

April 27th 2016
Now not Then
Jacobin   **Series of two, 79**
Robert Ewing

246

June 21st 2016
I'm unselfish; you're selfish
Robert Ewing   Series of one, 81-82

May 25th 2016
Is equality a right?
maoliosa   Series of four, 83-84
Robert Ewing
O'Murchú
Robert Ewing to O'Murchú

June 15th 2016
Irish poets learn your trade
Dozey   Series of four, 85-86
Robert Ewing to Dozey
Robert Ewing /Robert Ewing

June 15th 2016
Imagine
Robert Ewing /Robert Ewing   Series of two, 87

June 16th 2016
Stalin/out
Robert Ewing /Robert Ewing   Series of two, 89-92

August 9th 2016
Culture is ethics not just aesthetics
Darina Daly   Series of three, 93-94
totus tuus
Robert Ewing

August 29th 2016
New Constituti-on/off
Robert Ewing /Robert Ewing   Series of two, 95-99

August 14th 2016

Culture bids can be about change, not money

Robert Ewing   Series of one, 101

July 5th 2016

Judicial disappointments

dora at follyfoot   Series of eight, 111-115

dogears

David langwallner

Robert Ewing

Village Ed to dogears

Robert Ewing to dora at follyfoot

Robert Ewing to Village Ed

Robert Ewing to David langwallner

December 15th 2016

Judging the Guards

tad greenway   Series of five, 117-119

Lucy Byrne

JimJam

Robert Ewing

Robert Ewing to Lucy Byrne

March 2nd 2017

Extremism has become normal

Robert Ewing   Series of three, 121-122

Helen Collins

Robert Ewing

January 24th 2017

Adventures in British Imperialism

John Taurus   Series of four, 123-125

Robert Ewing to John Taurus

Robert Ewing /Robert Ewing

November 13th 2017
How do the poor die?
Robert Ewing /Robert Ewing   **Series of two, 145-146**

November 28th 2017
Lowry and Sinclair
Robert Ewing /Robert Ewing   **Series of five, 157-161**
Robert Ewing /Robert Ewing /Robert Ewing

December 19th 2017
The Rule of Law in Ireland, end 2017
Helen Collins   **Series of one, 180**

February 26th 2016
The March comments to *Election 2016*   **Series of two:**
Padraictheplasterer   **108**
Gunning for ideas   **105**